The Stevia Story

A tale of incredible sweetness & intrigue

by Linda Bonvie, Bill Bonvie
and Donna Gates

Foreword by James S. Turner,
author of "The Chemical Feast"

Excerpts on page 46 are reprinted with the permission of Simon & Schuster from *Who Will Tell The People* by William Greider. Copyright © 1992 by William Greider

The Stevia Story is written as an information resource and education guide for both professionals and nonprofessionals. It should not be used as a substitute for your physician's advice (although it is our hope that your physician is one who knows the importance of diet in healing and who has experience in treating Candida-Related Complex and other immune disorders). While we stand by the recommendations made in this book, you should make your decisions based on all the information at hand, knowing that you are the primary force in directing your own life and health.

ISBN: 0-9638458-1-0

Printed in the United States of America

B.E.D. Publications Co.
Atlanta, GA 30327

This book is dedicated to children everywhere in the hopes that they may be able to savor life's sweetness without having to suffer the adverse effects of consuming excessive sugar or artificial sweeteners.

TABLE OF CONTENTS

FOREWORD

Eat at Your Own Risk

by James S. Turner

Author of *The Chemical Feast* and *Making Your Own Baby Food*

Linda Bonvie called me first in April of 1992. Her diligent reporting on methyl bromide, a particularly noxious poison the FDA allows processors to apply to food, had, quite incidentally, led her to become interested in the subject of brominated vegetable oil (BVO), an additive manufacturers use in soft drinks. BVO keeps orange and other citrus sodas from clouding up in the bottle. It also caused heart damage in 1960s animal studies. Linda could get no BVO information from the FDA until one day an FDA official called her and said that while moving her desk she had found a 21-year-old letter "from Jim Turner to the FDA about BVO." She faxed the letter to Linda, who called me that day.

The letter concerned a lawsuit that Mike Jacobson, executive director of the Center for Science in the Public Interest (CSPI), and I brought against the FDA shortly after I wrote *The Chemical Feast: The Nader Report on the Food and Drug Administration* in 1970. We had filed suit to stop the use of BVO. The judge did not, as we asked, prohibit BVO use unless further studies established its safety. Instead he allowed the FDA to set up a new "interim" additive category. He envisioned a list of additives not yet established as safe but given time (two years for BVO) to meet the requirements of the law. Now, over 20 years later, BVO remains on the list and untested.

During the BVO suit, I saw the aspartame scandal develop. An FDA task force found numerous violations of sound scientific practice in studies designed to support aspartame approval. The FDA seized and sealed all research records, officially requested a grand jury investigation, and convened a public board of inquiry (PBOI) to review the studies. The PBOI ruled against marketing aspartame. However, the U.S. attorney ignored the grand jury request and let the statute of limitations run out. Supposedly sealed records turned up altered in a

1

pro-aspartame researcher's possession. A newly (Reagan) appointed FDA commissioner approved aspartame over the objections of his own advisors.

Aspartame, best known as NutraSweet, underscores two points about American food: FDA rules do not ensure safe food, and people want sweet tastes. In this book, Donna Gates and Linda and Bill Bonvie point out FDA weaknesses and identify a useful alternative. The FDA's clean bill of health for NutraSweet and guarded approval for other manufactured sugar alternatives, combined with its effort to suppress stevia, puts every consumer on notice —- you're on your own. As George Will once said, "The three least credible lines in English are: 'Yes I'll respect you in the morning,' 'The check is in the mail,' and 'I'm from the government and I'm here to help.'" Based on its record, FDA's job is to help food manufacturers, not consumers.

The American Dietetic Association's position on candidiasis further complicates the issue for consumers. This organization, with 50,000 members trained to provide consumers with dietary guidance, asserts that candidiasis does not exist. (It officially disciplined at least one member who it said suggested otherwise.) It also received a grant from the NutraSweet company to support its nutrition-information telephone line. In this environment of entwined relationships between food regulators, food manufacturers and the purveyors of food information to the public, consumers need to look to other sources for help. With this book, Donna Gates and the Bonvies provide one such useful source.

James S. Turner
Washington, D.C.
July 1996

PREFACE
by Donna Gates

Many years ago, I began research into what became The Body Ecology Diet, a new way of eating that can help people recover their health and restore their immune systems. I found that the most common condition shared by those who are ill is a condition known as candidiasis (also known as "candida"), an internal yeast overgrowth that thrives on sugar.

In a healthy body, a small amount of yeast is always present in our digestive tracts. The problems begin when this yeast (a type of fungus) gets out of balance and begins to take over the body, even inhibiting the function of key organs. Today we have a population raised largely on a combination of antibiotics, cortisone, steroids, birth-control pills and a broad range of other drugs. Antibiotics, in particular, devastate the body's natural immune system by destroying the beneficial bacteria that normally compete with the yeast for living space. The result is that candida has reached epidemic proportions. Typically, candida is a precursor to a wide range of progressive immune disorders, ranging from the deadly (AIDS, various cancers) to the debilitating (chronic fatigue syndrome, memory loss) to the merely annoying (vaginal itch, athlete's foot, jock itch).

Diagnosis is difficult because the symptoms are so diverse. But the real difficulty lies in finding a genuine cure rather than simply a way to suppress the symptoms. Though several expensive pharmaceutical products are available for that purpose, I knew that a lasting cure had to come from within the body itself. The internal healing capacity of the body had to be restored. That was the origin of The Body Ecology Diet.

Early on, it became clear that I was missing one key ingredient if this diet was to succeed: a viable sugar substitute. Because I knew the many harmful side effects of the pharmaceutical sweeteners (aspartame, saccharin), I began my search for a natural substitute. However, every sweetener that I found fed the yeast — fructose, honey, rice syrup, barley malt, even the sugar in fruit, grains and milk (lactose). The fungus thrived on them all.

3

For dietary purposes, it was essential that I find an appropriate sweetener. Even if people know that sugar feeds their candida, they still want sweets. From my study of Chinese medicine, I knew that the desire for sweetness is natural, just like the desire for other tastes (salty, sour, bitter and pungent). So rather than change human nature, I began looking for nature's answer to the problem. That's when I discovered stevia.

My first encounter with stevia was not encouraging. A popular multilevel marketing firm was selling stevia as one component of a face mask. A dark-green stevia syrup (derived from stevia leaves) was packaged with a small bottle of clay. The instructions recommended that the clay be blended with the stevia syrup and applied to the face, but it was the syrup's potential as a sweetener that interested me. It proved to be intensely sweet with a strong licorice-like aftertaste. Later I learned that I had used far too much — a common mistake. Fortunately, a much more tasty version of stevia was available.

Atlanta is now my home, but during this time I was living in Washington, D.C. Over dinner with two dear friends from the Chinese embassy, I mentioned my frustrating search. To my surprise, several weeks later, my friends presented me with an envelope containing a fluffy white powder that they had requested from a Chinese University. I found myself holding a sample of stevioside crystals extracted from Chinese-grown stevia plants using award-winning Japanese technology. The Japanese import enormous amounts of stevia from China to satisfy their world-famous taste for sweets. In a joint venture with the Chinese, they had developed a special technology to extract stevia's super-sweet crystals from the plant, leaving behind the licorice-tasting residue and creating a concentrated powder that, by weight, is 200 to 300 times sweeter than sugar.

I was thrilled. Here was a widely used, totally natural sweetener that had almost no calories, actually inhibited tooth decay and would not feed yeast. I began experimenting with it — baking with it, adding it to beverages and making stevia-flavored desserts. Many of those I counsel began to use it in place of sugar. They could now enjoy a sweet taste and still get rid of their candida. Soon thereafter, I arranged for delivery of a large amount of stevia, both for my personal use and to make available to clients.

4

Then a very curious thing happened. The Food and Drug Administration (FDA) labeled stevia an "unsafe food additive" and issued an alert blocking the importation of any more stevia into the United States. This seemed a really peculiar development. After all, not that many people knew about stevia and it was sold almost solely in health food stores. As the months rolled by, I noticed that the health food stores, knowing of the ban, continued to sell stevia quite openly. It moved quickly off the shelves as loyal customers bought the last available supplies. Then it was gone.

During this time, I did an enormous amount of research. First, I used a Freedom of Information Act request to ensure that I had all the information on stevia then in the hands of the FDA. No indication of any ill effects appeared anywhere in any of the literature, nor in other reports that I found independently. Plus, I was using it regularly as were many people I knew. Not only was no one adversely affected; everyone loved it. Most importantly, my friends who suffered from candida were overjoyed to finally have a sweetener they could use.

It was about this time that I moved to Atlanta and decided to take a stand. The FDA had by then succeeded in stonewalling the marketing of stevia by refusing to consider petitions that sought to have it officially placed on the generally recognized as safe, or "GRAS" list. That put stevia supporters in a classic "Catch-22" position, since no one would be willing to invest the millions of dollars (and the years of effort) required to move stevia through the FDA approval process as a food additive. That's because, unlike aspartame (sold as "NutraSweet" and "Equal"), stevia is an herb and not a patentable pharmaceutical product. So even if anyone could succeed in getting it approved as a food additive, they could not (unlike NutraSweet's manufacturer) exclude everyone else from the market while recovering their costs of moving it through the FDA bureaucracy. Once stevia was approved as an additive (if ever it was), then anyone could import it. Economists call that a "free rider" problem: one person pays the costs of obtaining the approval and then everyone else rides along on their approval — for free. Financially, it would not be a sound investment — a fact obvious to the FDA.

Taking the offensive, I began talking to others. The first was Dr. Robert Atkins, a cardiologist who has written seven popular books on diet and nutrition and is best known for his advocacy of a high-protein, low-carbohydrate diet. When I introduced Dr. Atkins to stevia, he immediately saw its value and used his widely read newsletter, Health Revelations, to recommend its use. He also made it available through his Manhattan-based Atkins Center for Complementary Medicine. Based on his instructions, his staff dietitian developed several delicious stevia-sweetened ice-cream recipes.

I also approached Dr. Julian Whitaker, another best-selling author and founder of the Whitaker Wellness Center. Though Atkins and Whitaker disagree in some of their approaches to diet and nutrition, both recommend stevia. Whitaker used his Health & Healing newsletter to tout stevia to almost a half-million subscribers. With their help, very quickly, hundreds of thousands of people learned about stevia.

Dr. Andrew Weil also recommended stevia in his widely read column for Natural Health magazine. At trade expos, I met with natural foods manufacturers who were eager to embrace stevia as a sweetener but were fearful of the FDA. I also spoke to manufacturers (such as ice-cream maker Ben Cohen of Ben & Jerry's) who very much wanted to sell a sugar-free, non-aspartame product — but who could not risk running afoul of the FDA. Despite concerns about possible repercussions, everyone said they were willing to help. Body Ecology's phone began to ring off the hook. A grass-roots movement had begun.

About this time, the FDA made a serious mistake: it attempted to take control of dietary supplements and herbal products. If the agency had gotten its way, you could not even purchase Vitamin C without a doctor's prescription. Congress had never seen such a response from a public unwilling to give up its rights. Based on that uproar, even outrage, the lawmakers moved quickly to halt this grab for power. As never before in its history, the natural foods industry became united.

Based on continued pressure from the public, from the natural foods industry and from the American Herbal Products Association, Congress passed the Dietary Supplement Health and Education Act. As a result of that, along with a subsequent "premarket notification" by Sunrider International (to introduce stevia as a dietary supplement), in September 1995 the FDA conditionally lifted its import ban on stevia.

So stevia began to flow back into the United States. Not, mind you, as a sweetener, but only when labeled as a dietary supplement. Its natural sweetening qualities, the FDA warned, would still be considered a "technical effect," and, thus — even now — should not be mentioned. While the natural foods industry was encouraged by the lifting of the import ban, few have wanted to attract the attention of the FDA by including stevia in their products and advertising it for what it is — a sweetener.

Some producers are simply going underground, hoping that common sense and the public interest will one day prevail at the FDA. For instance, several producers continue to use stevia as a sweetener but they've changed their ingredients label to read "natural flavors" instead of stevia. At Body Ecology, we have designed and produced several products using stevia, including "Eco Renew," a delicious raspberry-flavored sweet chewable Probiotic that is loved by both adults and children.

I know all this must sound bizarre. It is. I still cannot believe that, as this book goes to press, a natural, low-calorie, safe-for-diabetics, nonpharmaceutical sweetener that is widely used in other countries, including Japan (whose Ministry of Health is notoriously more strict than the FDA), cannot be openly sold as a sweetener in this country. After reading this book, you will need to draw your own conclusions regarding just why that is. As for me, my focus remains on how best to empower people to heal themselves.

Although it was never my intention to be in the stevia business, my discovery of the many benefits of stevia has proven to be providential in another respect because, without the resulting revenues, Body Ecology's grass-roots effort could not have been sustained — and you would not now be reading this book. So consider yourself part of a grass-roots conspiracy in the best

Jeffersonian tradition. Just like everyone else, the government makes mistakes from time to time. This is one of those times. We've all been taught that the legitimacy of our political system is based on the premise that it responds to the will of those who participate in it. I just never thought I would be called upon to participate in quite this way. It's been exciting, occasionally worrisome, always interesting and hugely gratifying.

But the job is not yet over. We still need your help. Because stevia remains in legal limbo, food manufacturers remain resistant to using it in products. If we can convince you after reading this book that stevia is your sweetener of choice, please join us in our efforts to make stevia widely available. What can you do? Use it yourself. Tell others, especially those with children. Request that your grocer stock stevia-sweetened foods. Write to your members of Congress. Write the FDA. Stop using aspartame products and urge others to cease.

Our health would be greatly enhanced if only we reduce the amount of sugar we consume...especially refined sugar. That's easy to do. By blending stevia with high-quality, healthier sugars (mineral-rich natural sugars such as molasses, barley malt, rice syrup, honey), we can still have delicious low-sugar treats. Note, however, that foods baked with stevia do not rise as much as those baked with sugar. Experiment to find the right combination of stevia (for sweetness) and sugar (for the rising effect) to create delicious low-sugar desserts. Once stevia becomes more widely available, I am confident that our creative food technicians and chefs here in America (as in Japan) will apply their ingenuity to bring us a range of delicious stevia-sweetened products.

If you are a chef or a professional baker, experiment with stevia. Here in Atlanta, chefs have created delicious beverages, baked goods (pies, cakes, cookies), sorbets, ice creams, puddings, even different flavors of stevia-sweetened mousse. You can take pride in joining those who are working to offer Americans healthier, higher quality sweets — without sacrificing anything to taste. Please share those recipes with us. We'll try them too, and credit you for those we include in the next edition.

With stevia now (we hope) poised for broader use and even full FDA acceptance, we are seeing the beginnings of what might be predicted: various qualities of stevia are finding their way onto the shelves. In part, this is a natural off-shoot of the extraction technology which can be adjusted to produce stevia powder that is either 95% or 55% stevioside crystals. In other cases, retailers are simply cutting the stevia with other ingredients, reducing both its strength and purity, or selling less refined versions. So when you choose a stevia supplement, make certain you know just what it is you're buying.

I know and, more importantly, those I counsel know from their own experience that stevia can play a role in helping people recover their health and restore their immune system. With our health-care industry now consuming 15 cents out of every dollar spent by American households, we must find better, more affordable ways to care for ourselves. Most importantly, our children must be taught that preventive health-care practices are their best possible health-care investment. We have been blessed with bodies that are designed both for health and for natural healing. We simply need to become wiser about how to tune into nature's own healing power.

Which brings me to this book, another key component of the stevia awareness campaign. I first became acquainted with Linda and Bill Bonvie when Linda interviewed me for a story she and Bill were writing on stevia. Her many months of research really impressed me. Their article later appeared in New Age Journal, along with a photo of our Body Ecology stevia. She had gotten my name from Julian Whitaker's newsletter.

After spending the better part of a year interviewing FDA personnel, poring over the worldwide research and talking to anyone who knew anything about stevia, it was clear that the Bonvies and I should collaborate on this latest step in advancing this benign conspiracy to bring you a safe and healthful sweetener. I hope that the resulting product — The Stevia Story - A Tale of Incredible Sweetness and Intrigue — is one that you will find enlightening and entertaining. I also hope it helps you make your personal transition to health and wholeness.

If you have any questions, or encounter any difficulties locating this great "dietary supplement," just call us at Body Ecology:

1-800-4STEVIA.

ABOUT THE AUTHORS

Linda and Bill Bonvie

Linda and Bill Bonvie are a New Jersey-based sister/brother writing team specializing in health/environmental issues. In addition to chronicling the stevia saga (originally for New Age Journal magazine), their achievements include breaking the story on the spraying of international airline flights with a hazardous pesticide. This led to actions by both the U.S. Environmental Protection Agency and the U.S. Department of Transportation that eventually persuaded many of the countries involved to abandon their requirements for such spraying.

The Bonvies have also published articles on such topics as the hazards accompanying the widespread use of the deadly fumigant methyl bromide, and the link between Gulf War Syndrome and the condition known as multiple chemical sensitivity. Their articles have appeared in a number of magazines and many major newspapers, including *The Philadelphia Inquirer, St. Louis Post-Dispatch, Cleveland Plain-Dealer and The Chicago Tribune*.

Donna Gates

Donna Gates is a nutritional consultant and an expert on candidiasis and related immune disorders. She has conducted extensive research on how these debilitating conditions affect the body, mind, and spirit. She developed the Body Ecology Diet and tested it on many different people who have all improved their health by following the basic principles of the Diet. She has studied with the top macrobiotic teachers and graduated from Lima Osawa's cooking academy in Japan. She holds an M.Ed. in Counseling from Loyola University and a B.S. in Early Childhood Development from the University of Georgia.

CHAPTER 1
Take another look at your sweetener

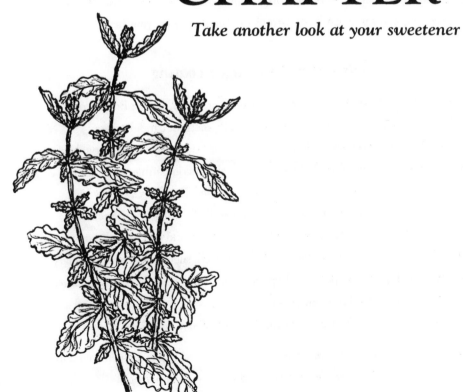

Look up the word "sweet" in the dictionary, and one of the definitions you'll find is "pleasing or agreeable." That definition, however, applies only in one sense to the conventional sweeteners currently available, whether natural or artificial. For while all may be "pleasing" to the taste, they can hardly be described as "agreeable" in their effects on the body.

To begin with there are the "natural" ones — sugar, or sucrose (white sugar plus maple, turbinado and raw sugar), honey, and corn syrup (including high fructose corn syrup, an industrial-strength variety treated with enzymes to intensify sweetness). Then there are the test-tube types, consisting mainly of aspartame (NutraSweet, Equal), saccharin, and acesulfame K (Sunett, Sweet One). Chances are, unless you're weight-conscious or diabetic — or have been introduced to *The Body Ecology Diet* — you've stuck with sugar, though you may also consume commercial products containing high fructose corn syrup. Otherwise, you've most likely opted for one or more of the artificial alternatives on the premise (and the promise) that it will help you stay trim and healthy.

In reality, however, none of the conventional sweeteners are particularly good for you, and some can be disastrous in their effects on your health.

Distress with a sugar coating

One of the problems with sugar (as discussed at length in *The Body Ecology Diet*) is its tendency to contribute to the development of candidiasis or Candida Related Complex, a prevalent condition caused by an overgrowth of the yeast known as candida albicans. Sugar is also incompatible with many other food ingredients, i.e. protein and starches (see The Body Ecology Diet chapter on food combining) — even in supposedly 'healthy' forms such as honey or maple syrup — often resulting in excess gas and digestive discomfort. Critics link sugar to a host of other ailments as well, such as diabetes, coronary heart disease, high blood pressure, hypoglycemia, yeast infections and inflammatory bowel disease. These medical disadvantages are in addition to sugar's more familiar ones, such as contributing to tooth decay and obesity.

The market for synthetic sweeteners has been fueled largely by personal concerns about sugar's high caloric content and its impact on diabetes.

Pharmaceutical sweeteners (which are really what these products are) have become widely available in soft drinks, in snack foods and desserts, as well as in packet forms (such as "Equal" and "Sweet 'N Low"). Despite their manufacturers' claims to the contrary, none of these products can be said to possess a 'clean bill of health.'

The synthetic picture — How sweet it isn't

The U.S. Food and Drug Administration (FDA) acknowledges as much in the case of saccharin, which comes with a label warning that it has caused cancer in laboratory animals. In fact, saccharin was allowed to remain on the market by virtue of a special act of Congress, whereas cyclamates, another type of chemical sweetener, were banned as a suspected carcinogen in 1970 — a ban that the Calorie Control Council has petitioned to have overturned.

Aspartame, by contrast, has no warnings attached to it other than one regarding its use by anyone with phenylketonuria (PKU), a rare condition that afflicts only one in 15,000 Americans. Uninformed consumers thus assume that they can use it with impunity, ingesting it directly or as a sweetener in more than 1,000 products (which often give scant indication that they contain it). As its use has accelerated, however, so, too, have the health complaints associated with it, along with the concerns raised by an increasingly vocal alliance of medical experts and activists.

Discovered in 1965 in the course of ulcer-drug research, aspartame is comprised of phenylalanine, aspartic acid and methanol, or wood alcohol (which, when ingested, breaks down into formaldehyde). Aspartame has been the prime suspect for a variety of symptoms chronicled in thousands of consumer complaints to the FDA and the Dallas-based Aspartame Consumer Safety Network. These include gastrointestinal problems, headaches, rashes, depression, seizures, memory loss, blurred vision, blindness, slurred speech and other neurological disorders.

Because it is a neurotransmitter — one of a class of chemicals manufactured and used by the brain — the aspartic acid in the aspartame is also believed by some experts to cause brain lesions by literally exciting some brain cells to

15

death — especially in children and in older people whose blood-brain barrier may not be fully functional. The sweetener is likewise considered a possible factor in the development of certain neurodegenerative diseases and brain tumors, according to Dr. Russell Blaylock, an aspartame critic and associate professor of neurosurgery at the Medical University of Mississippi.

Indications that aspartame produced brain tumors in laboratory rats caused some scientific advisors to the FDA to recommend that it not be approved. Their opinions were overridden by then-FDA Commissioner Author Hull Hayes, a Reagan appointee, who gave a green light to its various uses at the beginning of the 1980s, during the deregulatory heyday of the first Reagan Administration. Since then, however, there has taken place what the Community Nutrition Institute of Washington, D.C., describes as a "dramatic and sustained increase in the incidence of brain tumors in the United States." The possibility that this increase, along with a shift toward greater malignancy of such tumors, may be linked to aspartame use was raised in the November 1996 issue of *The Journal of Neuropathology and Experimental Neurology* by Dr. John Olney and other scientists from the Washington University School of Medicine in St. Louis.

According to their report, "there are three major criteria that are usually involved in evaluating the potential of an environmental agent to behave as a human carcinogen: (a) Does the agent have in vitro mutagenic potential? (b) Do experimental animals show an increased incidence of specific types of cancer when exposed to the agent? (c) Do humans show an increased incidence of the same types of cancer when exposed to the agent? Based on the limited evidence available, aspartame appears to meet all three criteria."

While the NutraSweet Company, with support from the FDA, has gone to considerable lengths to proclaim the safety and widespread acceptance of its product, critics insist that such confidence is ill-founded, based on highly questionable if not corrupt research. They point to charges by an FDA task force that cast serious doubt on the integrity of tests performed on aspartame by G.D. Searle, then NutraSweet's parent company — misgivings swept aside by Commissioner Hayes after Donald Rumsfeld, an influential member of the Nixon and Ford administrations, was named chairman of Searle. "It was

16

approved in a completely nefarious, completely unacceptable manner," says Washington D.C. attorney James S. Turner, author of the landmark book, *The Chemical Feast*. "It appears that Hayes was clearly placed in there for the purpose of getting this thing approved." There are about 20 studies that should be redone, Turner maintains, which he believes will demonstrate harm from aspartame.

One might assume, of course that such harm is offset by the purported benefits of aspartame, such as weight loss. But that's not necessarily the case. Studies cited by Dr. Blaylock and other medical experts show that the low-calorie sweetener actually tends to stimulate the appetite and, thus, may be a contributing factor in the marked increase in obesity among Americans, an increase that has coincided precisely with the period during which aspartame has been promoted as a way to help people control their weight.

Finally, there's the latest in synthetic sweeteners, Acesulfame K (marketed as Sunett and Sweet One), which requires neither a health warning nor an information statement on its product labels. At first blush, you might conclude that at last we have some good news about a sugar substitute — until you hear what the Center for Science in the Public Interest (CSPI) thinks of this alleged advance. Claiming that Acesulfame K "causes cancer and should not have been approved by the Food and Drug Administration," CSPI first objected a decade ago to the FDA allowing the product on the market. More recently, it reacted to consideration of Acesulfame K as a soft-drink sweetener by calling for the product to be banned until such time as it can be retested. CSPI also asked that any new tests be performed by the National Toxicology Program. "There are indications that it might be carcinogenic," noted Dr. David Rall, former NTP director and one of eight experts whose conclusions were submitted by CSPI to support its position.

In an earlier statement, CSPI Executive Director Michael Jacobson said he was "shocked that FDA would approve the use of a chemical that caused such obvious problems in two studies on laboratory rats." The studies in question, submitted by Sunett's manufacturer, Hoechst AG of Frankfurt, Germany, and its U.S. subsidiary, Hoechst Celanese Corp. of Somerville, N.J., found that the substance caused lung tumors in both male and female rats, premature deaths

17

among male rats, and mammary gland tumors in a second group. Using established cancer principles, those results make a strong case that Acesulfame K causes cancer, according to Lisa Lefferts, a former CSPI staff scientist.

But if that's true, how did such findings clear the FDA? Through the agency's use of "statistical tricks to make the tumors go away," contended Jacobson, who accused the FDA of "bending over backwards to help industry. It's not good science," he declared "and it's not good public health."

Not that such objections carry weight with the FDA, which in early 1992 denied CSPI requests both for a stay of its final ruling on Acesulfame K and for a hearing on its arguments, stating that "the agency has concluded that the objections do not raise issues of material fact that justify granting a hearing or revoking the regulation." In another ruling in December, 1994, the regulators approved a number of new uses for the additive, allowing it in yogurt products, frozen and refrigerated desserts, sweet sauces, toppings and syrups, baked goods and baking mixes.

Still, the FDA can't quite bring itself to recommend the kind of indulgence in Acesulfame K that might be encouraged by its lack of calories. The agency has established "an acceptable daily intake" of 900 milligrams per person per day. But while its calculations place the estimated daily intake from combined uses at 180 mg per day — "well below the acceptable daily intake" — actual consumption can easily be many times that amount. A single packet of Sweet One, for instance, contains 50 mg of Acesulfame K, and the substance can already be found in a substantial number of products, including major brands of puddings, chewing and bubble gums, flavored coffees, candy, breath mints, cough drops, and nutrition supplements. In addition, the recommended intake is geared to an "average" person weighing 132 pounds, according to an FDA source, indicating that someone weighing less — a 100-pound woman, for example — might have an even lower "acceptable" intake.

When Acesulfame K was first approved, Jacobson observed that "such controversies put the entire processed food supply under a cloud of doubt." It was also his feeling that "the public is waiting for an artificial sweetener that is unquestionably safe," but "unfortunately, this isn't it."

The answer that's been there all along

While the American public has waited in vain for a safe artificial sweetener to be developed, citizens of certain other countries have for years — in some cases, for centuries — enjoyed a safe, natural sweetener that is virtually calorie-free and widely believed to offer a host of other health benefits as well. This miracle sweetener is a South American herb called Stevia rebaudiana Bertoni — commonly known simply as stevia. Estimated to be some 150 to 400 times sweeter than sugar, stevia, after years of being kept from U.S. consumers, is at last on the verge of becoming the ideal answer to their 'sweet dreams.'

Why most Americans are only now finding out about stevia — and why it has been such an uphill struggle to make it available in the U.S. — is part of the story told in this book. It's a tale that offers a disturbing commentary on the relationship between government and business. But the story is exciting and heartening as well. What it reveals can help you enhance your health and well-being in spite of the FDA's misguided efforts.

CHAPTER 2

*Centuries-old appeal and
contemporary intrigue*

Medical researchers recently made some startling discoveries regarding an American Indian nation whose members today live on both sides of the U.S.-Mexican border. Those living north of the border were in extremely poor health; many were obese, while over a third suffered from diabetes. The ones on the Mexican side, however, were trim and robust, often still capable of hard physical work in their later years, and their rate of diabetes was less than a tenth that of their northern cousins.

When the researchers examined this disparity among people of similar genetic background, it didn't take long to identify an apparent cause. What they discovered was a correlation between the decline in health of tribal members living in the United States and their conversion to contemporary American dietary habits. Those north of the border had switched from customary native fare to processed foods containing refined sugar and flour, along with high levels of fat and low levels of fiber. Members of the tribe who remained in Mexico, however, had retained their traditional diet of unprocessed foods derived from natural sources, including desert cactus plants.

This finding suggests that what we commonly label "progress" is often delusionary, and that real advances in our lives may sometimes be a matter of embracing the old ways rather than equating advances in chemistry with advances in the human condition. This has become increasingly evident as science validates the efficacy of many so-called 'folk remedies' that were previously dismissed as quaint or ignorant.

With the growing worldwide emergence of stevia, we find another graphic example of this principle — along with a unique opportunity to benefit from the knowledge possessed by a centuries-old culture.

A powerfully sweet native tradition

There are those (FDA officials, for instance) who would characterize stevia as a "new" and "untested" commodity. True, it is something new to most U.S. consumers, in much the same way that the "New World" was new to the Spanish conquistadors who arrived on its shores during the 16th century. That world, however, was hardly new to its indigenous residents. And to those living in what is now northeastern Paraguay, neither was stevia — even way back then.

The Guarani Indians had known for centuries about the unique advantages of kaa he-e (a native term which translates as "sweet herb") — long before the invaders from the Old World were lured by the treasures of the New. These native people knew the leaves of the wild stevia shrub (a perennial indigenous to the Amambay Mountain region) to have a sweetening power unlike anything else; they commonly used the leaves to enhance the taste of bitter maté (a tea-like beverage) and medicinal potions, or simply chewed them for their sweet taste.[1] The widespread native use of stevia was chronicled by the Spaniards in historical documents preserved in the Paraguayan National Archives in Asuncion. Historians noted that indigenous peoples had been sweetening herbal teas with stevia leaves "since ancient times."[2] In due course, it was introduced to settlers. By the 1800s, daily stevia consumption had become well entrenched throughout the region — not just in Paraguay, but also in neighboring Brazil and Argentina.[3]

Like the discovery of America itself, however, credit for stevia's "discovery" goes to an Italian. In this case, the explorer was a botanist whose initial unfamiliarity with the region (along with his difficulty in locating the herb) caused him to believe that he had stumbled onto a "little-known" plant.

A New World "discovery"

Dr. Moises Santiago Bertoni, director of the College of Agriculture in Asuncion, first learned of what he described as "this very strange plant" from Indian guides while exploring Paraguay's eastern forests in 1887. This area was not the herb's native 'growing ground.' Consequently, Bertoni, by his own account, was initially "unable to find it." It was 12 years before he was presented with tangible evidence — a packet of stevia fragments and broken leaves received from a friend who had gotten them from the maté plantations in the northeast. He subsequently announced his discovery of the "new species" in a botanical journal published in Asuncion.

Bertoni named the "new" variety of the Stevia genus in honor of a Paraguayan chemist named Rebaudi who subsequently became the first to extract the plant's sweet constituent. "In placing in the mouth the smallest particle of any portion of the leaf or twig," Bertoni wrote, "one is surprised at the strange and extreme sweetness contained therein. A fragment of the leaf only a few square millimeters in size suffices to keep the mouth sweet for an hour; a few small leaves are sufficient to sweeten a strong cup of coffee or tea."

It wasn't until 1903, however, that Bertoni discovered the live plant, a gift from the parish priest of Villa San Pedro. The following year, as he recounted, "the appearance of the first flowers enabled me to make a complete study" — the publication of which appeared in December, 1905, after an interruption caused by a civil war. What he found was enough to convince him that "the sweetening power of kaa he-e is so superior to sugar that there is no need to wait for the results of analyses and cultures to affirm its economic advantage...the simplest test proves it."[4]

By 1913, Bertoni's earlier impression of what had now been dubbed Stevia rebaudiana Bertoni had undergone a change. What he had previously referred to as a "rare" and "little-known" plant had now become "famous" and "well-known." The botanist's initial misperception is explained by the Herb Research Foundation as being akin to that of a foreigner trying to find wild ginseng in the U.S., and coming to the erroneous conclusion that it is a rare plant when, in fact, it is widely prevalent — provided you know where to look. Further complicating the picture was the difficulty of traveling within Parguay during the late 1800s, entailing "an upriver journey of many days by steamship."[5]

This bit of historical trivia may seem inconsequential to us today. However, as we shall soon see, the question of whether stevia was obscure or common in that remote time and place has since emerged as a key factor in the decade-long battle to legalize its use in the United States.

Raising stevia — and the stakes

Bertoni's "discovery" was a turning point for stevia in one very real sense (other than being identified, analyzed and given a name). Whereas prior to

24

1900 it had grown only in the wild, with consumption limited to those having access to its natural habitat, it now became ripe for cultivation. In 1908, a ton of dried leaves was harvested, the very first stevia crop.[6] Before long, stevia plantations began springing up, a development that corresponded with a marked reduction in the plant's natural growth area due to the clearing of forests by timber interests and, to an extent, the removal of thousands of stevia plants for transplantation[7] (the growing of stevia from seed simply doesn't work). Consequently, its use began to increase dramatically, both in and beyond Latin America.

As word of this unique sweet herb began to spread, so, too, did interest in its potential as a marketable commodity. That, in turn, raised concerns within the business community. Stevia was first brought to the attention of the U.S. government in 1918 by a botanist for the U.S. Department of Agriculture who said he had learned about stevia while drinking maté and tasted it years later, finding it to have a "remarkable sweetness."

Three years later, stevia was presented to the USDA by American Trade Commissioner George S. Brady as a "new sugar plant with great commercial possibilities." Brady took note of its nontoxicity and its ability to be used in its natural state, with only drying and grinding required. He also conveyed the claims that it was "an ideal and safe sugar for diabetics." In a memo to the Latin American Division of the USDA, Brady further stated that he was "desirous of seeing it placed before any American companies liable to be interested, as it is very probable that it will be of great commercial importance."[8]

Stevia's commercial potential, however, was already known to others who were less than happy about it. In 1913, a report from the official public laboratory of Hamburg, Germany, noted that "specimens received are of the well-known plant which alarmed sugar producers some years ago."[9]

Rediscovered in Japan

While nothing came of this early show of interest in the United States, an event occurred in France in 1931 that would later prove significant. There, two chemists isolated the most prevalent of several compounds that give the stevia leaf its sweet taste, a pure white crystalline extract they named stevioside. One U.S. government researcher, Dr. Hewitt G. Fletcher, described this extract as "the sweetest natural product yet found," though adding, "It is natural to ask, 'of what use is stevioside?' The answer at this point is 'none.'"[10]

Within the next couple of decades, however, the enterprising Japanese had discovered just how useful stevioside really was. The Japanese either banned or strictly regulated artificial sweeteners during the 1960s, consistent with a popular movement away from allowing chemicals in the food supply. They soon discovered the ideal replacement for both sugar and its synthetic substitutes: refined stevia extracts.[11]

Originally introduced to Japan in 1970 by a consortium of food-product manufacturers, stevioside and other stevia products quickly caught on. By 1988, they reportedly represented approximately 41% of the market share of potently sweet substances consumed in Japan.[12] In addition to widespread use as a table-top sweetener, like the packets of saccharin ("Sweet-n-Low") and aspartame ("Equal") commonly found in the United States, stevia was also used by the Japanese to sweeten a variety of food products, including ice cream, bread, candies, pickles, seafood, vegetables, and soft drinks.

In addition to demonstrating stevia's nearly instant popularity in locales far removed from its native habitat, Japan's experience proved several other significant facts about this phenomenal plant: its adaptability and its safety. Adaptability was proven through the discovery that the plant could be grown throughout most of this temperate island nation, albeit under special hothouse conditions. Studies were even initiated to evaluate the substitution of stevia for rice under cultivation in some areas.[13] Stevia's safety was proven through extensive scientific testing, a matter we will discuss in Chapter 3.

The spread of the stevia phenomenon was not limited to Japan. Today it is also grown and used in approximately 10 other countries outside South America, including China, Germany, Malaysia, Israel and South Korea. Stevia might by now be entrenched in the United States as well, had it not been for a concerted effort to block its very entry.

The FDA says nay

By the mid-1980s, stevia's reputation had finally sparked the interest of various U.S. companies that were becoming aware of its potential commercial value, just as Commissioner Brady predicted some six decades earlier. With the addition of stevia to a number of popular brands of herbal tea (as a flavor enhancer), the remarkable ancient sweet herb of the Guarani Indians was at last poised to make a delayed debut in the American marketplace.

By this time, however, powerful market forces were at work, especially a huge artificial sweetener industry threatened by the appearance of a sweetener that was natural, virtually noncaloric and safe for diabetics — just as the sugar growers were alarmed over Bertoni's original "discovery." No sooner had stevia been introduced on the U.S. herbal scene that the FDA, just as quickly, launched an aggressive campaign to nip its emergence in the bud. A series of FDA-initiated actions against firms using stevia in their products (or buying it for that purpose) included embargoes, searches and seizures of warehouse and manufacturing facilities (complete with bevies of armed federal marshalls) and, to cap off the effort, a full-fledged "import alert" barring stevia shipments into the U.S.

Substantiated suspicions and spurned petitions

Just what prompted the FDA to intervene in the marketing of stevia, officials of the agency either cannot or will not say. Strong rumors persist that the catalyst was a "trade complaint" from a company that did not want stevia made available to consumers. As of this writing, no such complaint has yet surfaced that dates back to the launching of the FDA's campaign against stevia. However, an "anonymous" trade complaint submitted some time later is indeed on record, one that resulted in Celestial Seasonings, a Boulder, Colorado-based tea company, being forced to suspend its use of stevia in its popular line of herbal teas.

Lending further credence to suspicions that the FDA was acting at the behest of the artificial-sweetener industry are allegations that the NutraSweet Company was involved, charges that NutraSweet officials deny. However, one individual who was stopped from selling stevia products insists that an FDA representative specifically identified NutraSweet as the party that complained against his sale of an "untested natural sweetener."

None of this is acknowledged by the FDA as instrumental in its crackdown on stevia, which it characterizes as an "unsafe food additive." When closely examined, however, that claim appears to have nothing to back it up, while a substantial body of evidence to the contrary has been steadfastly ignored by FDA officials (as will be shown in an upcoming chapter).

Equally perverse has been the FDA's insistence that stevia is a relatively obscure herb about which little is known other than some "anecdotal" information. Despite the presentation of substantial historical data in two petitions seeking GRAS (generally recognized as safe) status for stevia (a designation to be discussed in detail later on), the FDA has held firm to its position that stevia's historical use was limited to "Indian ceremonies centuries ago," to quote the FDA's Dr. George Pauli. But that, says Pauli, "doesn't make (it) safe for general use in the food supply." In one of many self-contradictions, however, the FDA acknowledged in an import alert that "Stevia leaves...have been used throughout history."

The FDA even went so far as to claim that the petitions, submitted by the American Herbal Products Association and the Thomas J. Lipton Company, lacked sufficient data to enable them to be filed, a routine procedure that does not constitute approval, but does allow petitions to be viewed by the public. Overlooked was the fact that the agency, by its own admission, usually "perform(s) no in-depth prefiling review of actual data."[14]

The companies that introduced stevia in their products did so under a provision in federal law that allows for self-determination of GRAS status. They believe that stevia's long history of "common use in food" prior to 1958 (the year the FDA law took effect) and widespread use without any apparent adverse health effects provided them sufficient legal basis. By challenging that self-determination, what the FDA has done, in effect, is to dispute the validity of stevia's historical usage. This, in turn, is why Bertoni's divergent views of the plant as, first, "little-known" and , later, as "well-known" have become a matter of some importance to stevia's supporters.

28

A most peculiar paradox

By denying it official GRAS status, the FDA was able to place stevia in the "food additive" category, which requires that it undergo substantial scientific study prior to marketing (the kind of study already done in Japan but ignored by the FDA). The fact that stevia is a sweetener complicates the matter further, since the FDA tends to view any "new" sweetener as an additive with a particularly high potential for mass consumption, necessitating special scrutiny (although that attitude was relaxed in its rush to approve aspartame).

In 1994, however, passage of the Dietary Supplement Health and Education Act created an opportunity for stevia to enter the U.S. market despite the FDA's vehement opposition. Under that legislation, various vitamins, minerals, herbs or other botanicals not considered conventional foods or the sole item in a meal or diet may be marketed in the form of capsules, tablets, liquids, powders, or soft gels provided they are labeled "dietary supplements." Such supplements can no longer be classified by the FDA as "food additives" and need not be subjected to intensive safety testing.

The following year, stevia did indeed gain status as a dietary supplement after a 75-day "premarket notification" was submitted to the FDA. The agency could have challenged that, too (and still can, for that matter) by claiming adulteration based on inadequate safety information. Had it done so, however, the FDA would have borne the burden of proof for such a claim.

As a result, stevia at long last became legally available in the United States — but only in its limited form as a dietary supplement. Any other use (such as in teas or processed foods) continued to be prohibited. Also, the stevia saga took several odd turns.

For one thing, the FDA has adopted a totally nondefensible position by sanctioning the consumption of what it continues to label an "unsafe food additive." Its import alert, for instance, has remained in effect — only it has been revised to exclude stevia products "explicitly labeled as a dietary supplement."

Perhaps the strangest development, however, is in regard to stevia's role as a sweetener. The FDA has acknowledged that it considers stevia to be just that.

In fact, it describes the GRAS petitions it received (but never filed) as being for a "sweetener," even though neither petition calls for it to be used for this purpose. Indeed, the Lipton petition goes to great lengths to indicate that its intended use is only as a flavor, not as a sweetener.

One FDA official, Dr. David Hattan of the Division of Health Effects Evaluation, points to the difficulty inherent in making such a distinction because stevia is "potent enough as a sweetener so that even in the low concentrations (the petitioners hoped to use), it will have some effect of that nature."

Nevertheless, the FDA strictly prohibits stevia "supplements" from being labeled as sweeteners, or in any way described as having sweetening power, even while allowing supplements to feature health claims that have — as their labels must clearly state — "not been evaluated by the FDA."

In another era, this would have been great material for one of those absurd spoofs made famous by Gilbert and Sullivan: the most peculiar paradox that the word "sweet" must never to be used in labeling an herb described throughout its history as possessing "truly marvelous" sweetening power.

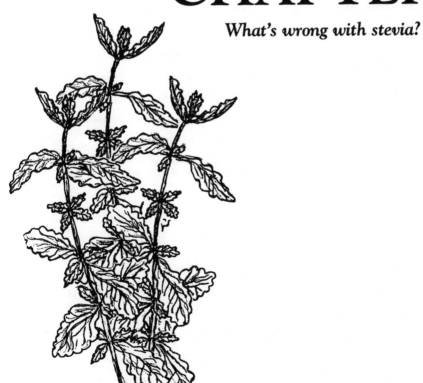

CHAPTER 3

What's wrong with stevia?

Where there's smoke, there's fire, goes an old saying. That's precisely the kind of thought that is apt to cross the minds of people reading about stevia for the first time: if it's as wonderful as you make it out to be, then why does the FDA insist on calling it an "unsafe food additive?" Surely, that kind of official label must mean there's <u>something</u> wrong with it. A federal agency, after all, would not be so frivolous as to stigmatize a product with claims that it couldn't back up, now, would it?

That may seem like a logical enough assumption — that is, until the FDA's "case" against the marketing of stevia is carefully analyzed. Closer examination suggests that the smoke raised by the FDA's objections is actually nothing more than a smoke screen, especially when one factors in the results of extensive scientific testing from abroad.

The three-decade-old study the FDA loves to quote

In what precise manner does the FDA consider stevia to be "unsafe?" Is it suspected of causing cancer in laboratory animals, like saccharin (which remains on the market nonetheless)? Has it been linked to the growth of brain tumors in rats, or to the development of holes in the brains of baby mice, the way aspartame has? Or is it believed by some medical experts to destroy brain cells through overstimulation, like aspartame? Have people developed health problems after using it, such as those that over seven thousand aspartame users have reported to the FDA, ranging from headaches to blindness?

The answer to all of the above is, quite simply, "no." There are a couple of possible effects, however, that FDA officials claim to be concerned about. They are concerned enough, in fact, to have gone to considerable lengths to protect U.S. consumers from stevia for more than a decade.

Their chief concern, it seems, is that stevia might act as (are you ready for this?) ... a contraceptive. To quote from an "information" sheet on stevia issued by the FDA's Center for Food Safety and Applied Nutrition, they are "concerned about this product because of two published scientific studies that suggest that the consumption of aqueous extracts of stevia reduces the fertility of female laboratory animals." The second page of that same information sheet

32

offers the agency's reassurance that aspartame "meets the safety standard for food additives of a 'reasonable certainty of no harm.'"

The more significant of the two studies cited — both prompted by rumors of stevia's use for contraceptive purposes by Indian women in South America — is one which took place in Uruguay nearly three decades ago, and whose conclusions researchers have been unable since to duplicate. The study was performed in 1968 by Professor Joseph Kuc, then a member of Purdue University's department of biochemistry, working with a faculty member of the University of the Republic in Montevideo.

While the results of the Kuc study would appear at first glance to bear out such rumors, closer examination raises doubts about the methods that were used, and how they apply to the typical way in which stevia is consumed. In fact, Kuc himself, although still standing by his findings of marked, relatively long-term reductions in the numbers of offspring born to female rats administered his stevia solution, acknowledges that those results aren't necessarily applicable to human consumption.

The Kuc study involved a very high concentration — ten milliliters of a dosage administered in about 20 minutes — of a concoction derived by drying to a powder and boiling not just the leaves, but material from the stevia plant that would not ordinarily be consumed. This liquid replaced the animals' drinking water, and was given at such a rate as to equate with a person drinking 2.5 quarts of liquid in less than half an hour.

The study also only utilized one dosage level. Typically, a biological effect (such as what Kuc reported) would be demonstrated by using a variety of doses to establish what is known as a dose-response relationship.[1]

Kuc acknowledges that the study "absolutely needs to be redone" (just as all research, in his view, needs to be "checked and rechecked" to determine whether it "stands the test of time"). He further concedes that this finding, in itself, does not constitute an important reason for keeping stevia off the U.S. market.[2]

"The topic of what is safe and is not safe is very pertinent, but it has to be looked at very carefully and in perspective; otherwise, people will be frightened about things they don't need to be frightened about, like the potato," says Kuc. "You eat potatoes, don't you, and you eat the peel. If you ate a pound of potato peel, you probably would die" from the toxins it contains. "During the war, people ate the peel, and they got very ill...but potatoes are nutritious; people have been eating them for a long time...I certainly wouldn't propose people not eat potatoes."

Kuc also notes something else: that effects in rats aren't necessarily experienced by people — as illustrated by the apparent lack of any correlation between the results of his rat research and birth rates among regular stevia consumers.[3] As pointed out in the Lipton petition to the FDA, "...if this reproductive effect in rats is real and can be extrapolated to humans, then one might suspect that there would be very few children in some regions of Paraguay."

That isn't to say that stevia might not have some "weak estrogenic properties," just as do many other plants, including a common example cited by the Lipton petitioners — the soybean.[4] But even the best available scientific evidence fails to make a case for stevia being a contraceptive with any potency — if, indeed, it is one at all.

Scraping the bottom of the research barrel

But hold on a moment. Wasn't there a second study dealing with stevia's supposed contraceptive effect?

Indeed there was. The particular study in question was one performed on female mice, the results of which were published in a Brazilian pharmacological journal in 1988 and later informally translated by an FDA employee familiar with Portuguese. The only problem is that, outside of the FDA, no one in the scientific community gives it credence.

The research at issue, according to one authority who analyzed it (Professor Mauro Alvarez of Brazil's State University of Maringa Foundation) "caused surprise with regard to the lack of information about the quantities that were administered and the preparation of the infusions, because mice, due to their low body weight, cannot receive high volumes intragastrically without suffering major stress." What's more, the study involved a small number of test animals and was "highly susceptible to external influences," he observed.[5]

The same study was characterized by Mark Blumenthal, editor of *Herbalgram* — a newsletter published jointly by the American Botanical Council and Herb Research Foundation — as "the kind of research which FDA would never accept if a petitioner was using it (as a basis for) his or her arguments." In his opinion, "The FDA would laugh them out of the room."

What's perhaps most interesting about the FDA's citation of these two studies, however, is that what it regards as a possibly harmful effect is just as apt to be viewed as a beneficial one. As the authors of the Lipton petition put it, "One would think that this effect would make stevia extract the perfect contraceptive agent — easy to consume, low toxicity, and effective long-term — and would be intensely pursued by pharmaceutical companies, the World Health Organization, etc. Obviously this has not happened (or if it has, then there was no effect), which casts further doubt on the validity of the data."[6]

How about this? — a hypothetical hypoglycemic effect

Maxwell Smart, the screwball secret agent of an old comic TV series, had a stock response whenever he was accused of offering some excuse or rationale that just wouldn't hold up — he would concoct an even more preposterous explanation invariably preceded by "How about this?"

In their apparent determination to prevent a potential stevia threat to the sweetener industry, officials at the FDA have taken a leaf from Maxwell Smart's book of the absurd with a "How about this?" of their own.

Just in case the public doesn't share their "concern" about stevia's possible contraceptive properties, how about this? Based on studies they've heard about through the South American grapevine — but have never seen — it's just possible that stevia might also be "unsafe" by virtue of having a hypothetical hypoglycemic effect on some individuals.

While it pushes the limits of credibility to think that a federal agency would stoop to anything so dubious, that is exactly what the FDA has done to buttress its campaign against stevia. Although its decisions are supposedly based on solid scientific findings, it has raised concerns in this case based on nothing more than rumor, innuendo, and vague speculation.

For instance, following passage of the Dietary Supplement Act, the FDA's Office of Premarket Approval, in reciting cautionary notes (to a firm that had filed notice of intent to market stevia as a supplement), asserted that "published studies raise concern over possible hypoglycemic effect. " When pressed for details, the FDA's Dr. Hattan conceded that the agency had never actually read the studies, which, according to Hattan were published "in a foreign language" in "small regional journals in South America." He may have been referring to studies mentioned in a safety review of stevia by Dr. A. Douglas Kinghorn, a University of Illinois pharmacognosy professor, who notes that these studies provide "some credence for the medicinal use of the plant in Paraguay" as a diabetes remedy (a subject to be covered in an upcoming chapter). Other studies, Kinghorn added, failed to detect any effect on carbohydrate metabolism.

"I don't think we've seen them," Hattan confessed. "We have attempted to get them, and thus far have not been successful." But what concerned the FDA, he claimed, was the theoretical possibility that stevia might cause blood sugar to drop too low in some hypoglycemic individuals. He added that while he thought there were some indications in the literature that stevia might have use as a "stabilizing, normalizing" factor in the condition, "it's not clear because we can't get access."[7]

The FDA's double standard

The FDA apparently is under no illusions about the quality of the stevia research it cites. Dr. Alan M. Rulis, of the FDA's Office of Premarket Approval, has acknowledged that the research wouldn't stand up to scrutiny if the situation were reversed and a petitioner had submitted it to the agency. But then, according to Rulis, "That's the case with all the data on stevia."[8] Or, as his colleague, Dr. Pauli, has stated, the studies at issue "are not the greatest science in the world, I will admit. But the fact is there just isn't a lot of good science on stevia. Certainly, we don't have any kind of data comparable to what we have for sweeteners used in food."[9]

As it turns out, however, there is quite a bit of "good science" on stevia that the FDA should be well aware of, since it's all detailed in those petitions that the agency has rejected as "inadequate" for filing. The significance of that scientific data becomes even more pointed when close comparisons are made with the data for "sweeteners used in food."

According to Rulis, for instance, the FDA has accumulated a "massive amount of information" on which it based its approval of aspartame — what he describes as "a portfolio of toxicological studies of very high quality" which were evaluated using a standard of "reasonable certainty of no harm." That's not to say, however, that all the information on aspartame was of a positive nature. "In any large data package, there will be adverse effects that are observed," he noted. "The question is, are those adverse effects mitigated by or contravened by other data of equal or better quality? I think in the case of aspartame, when all the data is taken together, the inescapable conclusion is you have a material here that is safe."

Where stevia is concerned, however, the picture suddenly changes. "When we see a study — even if it's a poor study — that implies the existence of an adverse effect that isn't resolved, we have to be concerned whether that effect really could happen," Rulis contended.

And what about the data that, in stevia's case, might tend to "mitigate or contravene" any adverse effects implied by admittedly "less-than-great science" — or by reports that FDA officials cite but haven't seen? When confronted with the question, Rulis couldn't answer, other than to make vague references to "the need to investigate that and have a discussion about that" and to find out "why our scientists have a concern that has not been erased."[10] Such comments leave little doubt that, at least in regard to stevia, the FDA has no qualms about utilizing a convenient double standard when it comes to evaluating health risks.

A verdict from the land of 'good science'

Stevia's safety record in Japan isn't only based on two decades of widespread use of the herb and its extracts there. (Japanese stevia consumption had already reached an estimated 170 metric tons in 1987 without a single report of an adverse reaction appearing in the scientific or medical literature.[11]) It is also based on a vast amount of research and testing by a nation with a formidable reputation for scientific know-how.

In one chronic toxicity study conducted in Japan, nearly 500 rats were fed stevia for up to two years, with the highest administered dosage representing 100 times the estimated daily human intake. According to Kinghorn, "this protracted and extensive investigation" led the researchers to conclude that no significant dose-related changes had occurred in growth, general appearance, hematological and blood biochemical findings, organ weights, and macroscopic or microscopic observations. As Kinghorn notes, "The results obtained are supportive of the safety of S. rebaudiana extracts, stevioside and rebaudioside A when consumed as sucrose substitutes by human populations."[12]

After another extensive Japanese study of subacute toxicity, it was concluded that feeding male and female rats up to seven percent stevioside for nearly two months produced no unfavorable toxic effects, nor did a similar study in South Korea, using aqueous extract containing 50 percent stevioside.

Results of further Japanese tests on both male and female laboratory rats directly refute the FDA's characterization of stevia as a possible contraceptive; neither of two studies produced any evidence of effects on fertility, or, for that matter, on either fetuses or offspring.

After subjecting stevia to full-fledged, lengthy, and comprehensive trials — both in the laboratory and in actual human use — one of the world's most scientifically advanced societies has embraced it. Meanwhile, the U.S. continues to keep stevia 'locked up' on suspicion of being "unsafe" (although at present in a kind of 'halfway house' reserved for dietary supplements), choosing to ignore the overwhelming evidence of its benign and beneficial character.

No sweet talk allowed

The Dietary Supplement Health and Education Act (DSHEA) of 1994 has done a bit more than open up to the public the availability of amino acids, vitamins, herbs, and minerals in the form of dietary supplements. It has also turned a few heads in conventional food companies as well.

Not only is DSHEA itself a perceived threat to "conventional" food products, but stevia, with its legendary sweetness, is a special concern. A recent trade publication carried an article by a prominent Washington food and drug attorney who is also counsel to the soft-drink industry. The article, "Could your food product be a dietary supplement?," cautions "every food processor (to evaluate) the potential competitive opportunities and threats posed by this new law."[1]

In a thinly disguised example of stevia sneaking through a supplement loophole, the lawyer warns about a botanical extract put in "little purple packets that a manufacturer wants to sell as a tabletop sweetener. Although the product has been widely used in Japan for 20 years without safety concerns, little toxicology data is available on the substance," he states, adding, "that product could potentially be sold today in those little purple packets if the product was labeled as a supplement with sweetening properties."[2]

Apparently the FDA took note of this cautionary tale. In its revised import alert (allowing stevia to enter the country as a dietary supplement) the agency made a special point of forbidding sweetness to be mentioned in the labeling of any stevia supplement. Any such reference would result in stevia's status reverting from that of an allowed product (dietary supplement) back to that of an "unsafe food additive."[3]

What about steviol?

Opponents of stevia, clutching for anything negative they might drum up to alarm consumers, occasionally mention steviol. Under certain laboratory conditions steviol can be created as a breakdown product from stevioside. It does not appear that the human body has this ability to metabolize steviol from stevioside. If we could metabolize stevioside into steviol, the question then would be, "Is steviol a mutagen?"

In the 1970s, the Japanese conducted a considerable amount of research to determine if stevia consumption produced any mutagenic or carcinogenic effects. The research showed no effects of that nature, leading the Japanese Ministry of Health and Welfare in 1977 to conclude that there was no cause for concern on this score.[1]

There are, however, a few studies suggesting that steviol could be a mutagen, but only under certain conditions. Some mutagens are carcinogens, some are not. The interesting thing about steviol is that there is not a shred of evidence to indicate it ever has been or even can be produced from stevia in a human being.

Dr. A. Douglas Kinghorn, professor of Pharmacognosy at the University of Illinois and one of the leading experts on stevia, feels it would be nice to resolve the steviol issue once and for all; however, he doesn't see it as a significant point. "I don't think it's that big a question mark because of the Japanese experience. They've been taking it for 20 years now and they've had multigenerations of humans using it. (To produce steviol) requires metabolic activation which may or may not happen," he points out.

Not only is this all "very conjectural," according to Dr. Kinghorn, but whether steviol is actually a mutagen or not is also still open to question. One lab, Kinghorn notes, found it to be "a very, very weak mutagen," while another found it not to be mutagenic at all. "We do have the evidence from the Japanese that stevioside is not carcinogenic. It hasn't been resolved whether steviol is produced in animals, let alone in humans."

CHAPTER 4

What's wrong with the FDA?

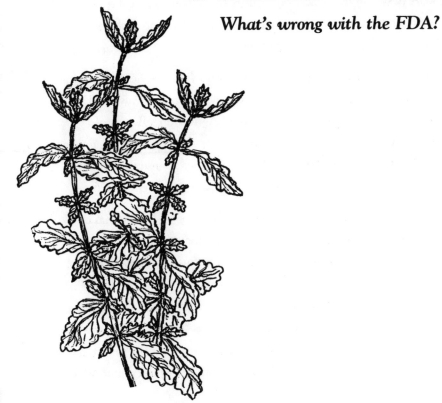

If the road to hell is paved with good intentions, so is the road to limbo. Perhaps no better illustration exists than the cautionary tale of the good intentions behind the FDA's origins, and how they have led to stevia being very cleverly — and very deliberately — cast into the bureaucratic limbo it now occupies.

Beyond stevia's significance for a society desperately seeking the benefits it has to offer, the FDA's treatment of this herb epitomizes the ambiguous relationship that often exists between government regulators and the regulated. On the one hand, the FDA's behavior appears to support its critics who claim that the agency meddles in the marketplace and discourages "competitiveness." On the other hand, this interference may trace its roots to influence wielded by commercial interests who want to see the FDA discourage competition.

Wiley and his Poison Squad

The massive, often cumbersome system of safety evaluation that characterizes today's FDA (a system that places on industry the burden of actual testing) bears little resemblance to the far simpler and more direct approach that marked the agency's inception a century ago.

It was Dr. Harvey Washington Wiley, a man who did not suffer food adulterators gladly, who first put a stop to some of the more rampant abuses in U.S. food production. As chief of the Department of Agriculture's Bureau of Chemistry for nearly 30 years — from 1883 to 1912 — Wiley led the crusade that spurred Congress to legislate on behalf of America's consumers, and thus came to be known as the father of the Pure Food and Drug Act of 1906.

A medical doctor with a Ph.D. in chemistry, Wiley based his findings on experiments that were perhaps a bit more germane than today's reliance on laboratory rats. His test animals were humans — Department of Agriculture volunteers who agreed to let Wiley monitor their consumption of a variety of additives over a five-year period. What Wiley concluded after carefully observing the reactions among those who became known as his "Poison Squad" was that many of the components of the American diet at that time were, in fact, downright dangerous. Possessing considerable skill as both writer and orator, Wiley

42

was then able to use the results of his research as a springboard for political action by arousing public sentiment against the adulterators.[1]

Wiley's original emphasis on empirical data gathering may seem primitive when contrasted with the sophisticated lab techniques now used for evaluating the safety of food additives, and which today's FDA uses in arriving at its findings. But perhaps that's part of what's wrong with the FDA. In the course of embracing scientific expertise, it lost the common-sense ability to recognize the value and validity of everyday experience as an indicator of what's safe and what isn't.

Inadmissible evidence in the court of expert opinion

A law, of course, is only as good as its enforcement. Like so many other legislative victories, the passage of the Pure Food Law of 1906 was only a beginning. It wasn't long before Wiley and its other supporters found themselves engaged in an uphill battle with those intent on weakening this particular law's clout.

One of the opposition's main maneuvers was to redirect the intent of the legislation by suggesting the use of guidelines rather than penalties for regulated industries. To this end, a practice emerged of convening get-togethers with industry representatives to discuss how the law might best be implemented through cooperative efforts.[2] Such meetings afforded large corporate interests an opportunity to work out various forms of compromise and to establish cozy working relationships with regulators, an opportunity available neither to consumers nor to smaller entrepreneurs, such as those engaged in the marketing of competing natural products.

The first major revision of the 1906 law was the Federal Food, Drug and Cosmetic Act of 1938. That act required that the safety of new drugs be proven prior to marketing. It wasn't until 20 years later that the law was expanded to shape the system currently in effect. Under the Food Additives Amendment of 1958, the food supply was divided into two general categories. The first category covered those commodities either generally recognized as safe (GRAS) for their intended uses or those given "prior sanction" either by the FDA or by the

U.S. Department of Agriculture. The other category encompassed everything else under the "food additives" heading. The FDA was then given a time frame in which to tackle such matters as rule implementation, designation of items on the GRAS list, and the approval of additives introduced before 1958, a process that took seven years. Also adopted during this period were the Delaney Clause, prohibiting carcinogens in processed food, and the Color Additives Amendment of 1960, regulating the use of food colors.

In reaching its decisions, the FDA has since relied both on scientific testing (performed by manufacturers) and on "expert" advisory panels. Both have frequently incurred the wrath of various critics. One industry spokesman, Washington, D.C., attorney Peter Barton Hutt (who served as FDA chief counsel during the early 1970s) has decried the agency's failure to approve more than a very small number of food additives introduced over the past 25 years, noting that the approval process is a "closed process within FDA, not subject to public scrutiny...and is solely within the control of the agency." By contrast, he characterizes the regulation of GRAS substances as an "enormous success" due to its "classic free market approach." He also contends that, in any event, no product in either category has "proved to present a public health hazard."[3]

Paradoxically, what allows Hutt to make such a claim is the very tendency that he considers one of the FDA's "major failings" — its inability to ever admit to making a wrong decision. Were the agency capable of doing so — and were it more receptive to the type of outside influence he advocates — it might have taken steps to reverse one of its decisions that has proved to present a public health hazard in the years since it was handed down: approval of the pharmaceutical sweetener aspartame.

The irony of the aspartame fiasco is that, unlike those self-determined GRAS substances, this chemical concoction was supposedly put through the rigid, comprehensive and time-consuming "expert" examination that the FDA demands before allowing a new additive to be introduced into the food supply. In retrospect, it's also revealing to note that aspartame was approved despite serious allegations of deception, and over the doubts of scientific advisers, due to what some believe was political pressure at the time from its corporate sponsors — not unlike a student from an influential family who's accused of fudging on his finals but manages to graduate nevertheless.

44

While it has become almost a reflex action on the FDA's part to dismiss as "unscientific" the thousands of complaints from consumers that have since been brought to its attention, the negative repercussions have found other ways of surfacing. For instance, many consumers have taken to venting their aspartame experiences on the Internet, responding to a query with hundreds of indignant and sometimes harrowing descriptions of incapacitating symptoms that disappear with the removal of aspartame from their diet.

Typical of these accounts:

"My legs used to hurt so bad I couldn't sleep at night, but when I suspected what it was and stopped using NutraSweet the pain went away. That stuff is POISON. I know because I've experienced it."

"I cannot eat anything containing aspartame as I quickly start to lose muscle control and tremble so that I can't even reliably hold a cup."

"I get deathly ill if I drink or eat anything with aspartame in it. I get nauseated, headaches and feel like I'm never going to get up again."

Perhaps most common are reports of people suffering excruciating migraines until giving up aspartame use. "For years I suffered from terrible, debilitating headaches that wouldn't respond to any medication," wrote one such complainant, who finally noticed that her headaches followed the consumption of a bowl of cereal sprinkled with aspartame. "That was the last time I used NutraSweet. That was the last time I had one of 'those' headaches."

"I suffered terrible headaches for three years," wrote another, who said a variety of medical treatments had proven ineffective. But after reading that NutraSweet might be a possible cause, "I stopped (consuming diet foods and soda containing it) and so did the headaches."

Others report even more alarming symptoms associated with aspartame use, such as bouts of blindness and seizures. One describes the result of convincing a friend, who had experienced epileptic seizures following a brain injury, to give up the diet products she consumed almost exclusively: "She took my advice, and her seizures almost completely disappeared. She can go for days now without one at all as opposed to one every half-hour. Her concentration and memory were like having a 'New Brain' (as she described it)."

45

In reviewing the many aspartame complaints — similar to those that the FDA has also logged (but effectively ignored) — one can't help but realize just how far the agency has strayed from Wiley's original approach to food safety that was based primarily on the effects of dietary components on consumers themselves. But then, the shunting aside of personal experience is something that has become all too characteristic of government agencies. As William Greider noted in his 1992 best-seller, *Who Will Tell the People: The Betrayal of American Democracy*:

> "On issue after issue, the public is belittled as self-indulgent or misinformed, incapable of grasping the larger complexities known to the policymakers and the circles of experts surrounding them... the public's side of the argument is described as 'emotional,' where-as those who govern are said to be making 'rational' or 'responsible' choices... The reality, of course, is that the ability to define what is or isn't 'rational' is itself laden with political self-interest, whether the definition comes from a corporate lobbyist or from a federal agency... Furthermore, the uncredentialed public sometimes 'knows' things before science does."[4]

Considering the degree of influence that corporate lobbyists now wield in Washington, the reconsideration of any decision in which industry has untold millions of dollars at stake might well be viewed as contrary to anyone's political self-interest. Nor would it serve the self-interest of a regulatory agency to admit that it was wrong, thereby potentially bringing other decisions into question. Thus, rather than acting on the most obvious indicators of harm, as Wiley would have done, today's FDA finds it more expedient to play the "expert" card, enabling it always to trump those lower ones of mere consumer experience.

A wrong turn away from the right of the consumer

The same type of bureaucratic arrogance can be seen in the case of the FDA's treatment of stevia, only in reverse. Now that stevia has been designated as "unsafe" — almost certainly, as a sacrificial sop to the politically powerful sweetener industry — the agency has insisted on stonewalling any and all evidence to the contrary. Once the decision has been made, neither practical experience nor scientific research are persuasive — no matter how ill-formed and groundless that decision might be. In the process, the FDA has also turned a deaf ear to the public's growing demand for a safe and virtually noncaloric natural alternative to sugar or to artificial sweeteners.

In essence, what's wrong with the FDA — as typified by the ascent of aspartame and the suppression of stevia — is that it forgot the chief lesson of its architect, Dr. Wiley: "the principle that the right of the consumer is the first thing to be considered."[5]

In so doing, it took a wrong turn away from its original purpose — and now harms the very consumers it was established to protect.

CHAPTER 5

A craving for sweets

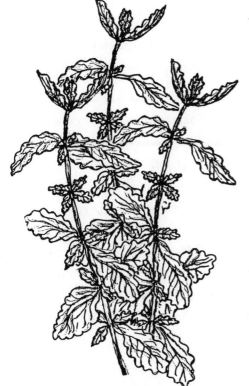

In the preceding chapters, we have told the story of stevia both from a historical and a contemporary perspective, covering the issues of its safety and availability. In so doing, we have also shown how these issues fit into a wider picture encompassing the politics of food, health and nutrition as practiced in the United States.

From this point on, our focus will be on the practical uses of stevia as an alternative to other available sweetening agents. Whether labeled disingenuously as a dietary supplement or by any other name, the fact remains that stevia tastes just as sweet as it did when first used centuries ago, and has remained every bit as beneficial.

The perfect natural sweetener

Have you ever had the desire that you absolutely, positively had to have something sweet? Unless that craving has sent you on chocolate bar or ice-cream binges, don't feel too bad. The desire for a sweet taste is one with which humans are born; in fact, mother's milk has more natural sugars than goat's or cow's milk.

What gets us into trouble is not the natural human tendency to crave something sweet, but rather what we use to satisfy that desire.

A craving for sweets is also a message the body sends to signal a need to open up and relax. Our bodies are engineered to maintain a proper balance of expansion and contraction. An excess of foods that are more contractive, such as salty foods and meats, as well as getting stressed or "uptight," will cause us to crave sweets, which are expansive. Such a desire is very often the body's way of trying to balance itself. However, it is not without its dangers. If you have a yeast condition, an immune disorder such as cancer, Epstein-Barr, candidiasis, herpes, AIDS, M.S., etc. sugar is definitely to be avoided. On the other hand, if you have a healthy body and a digestive tract teeming with wonderful, beneficial bacteria, then a moderate amount of sugar is not going to do the same damage. Synthetic sugar substitutes, as noted earlier, have other problems associated with them that should discourage their use in either case.

By introducing stevia into your diet, however, you can satisfy your sweet tooth without having to worry about the side effects. Since we don't live in Japan or a dozen or so other countries where stevia-sweetened food products are easily found — even products made by U.S. companies such as Sunkist and Nestle — it may take some initial effort to make the switch to stevia. But you'll soon find that the results are well worth the trouble.

Stevia is heat stable, which makes it ideal for baking (see chapter 7 for details on the different forms in which stevia is available), and can be used to make a variety of cookies and confections. It can also be used to enhance the flavor of other sweeteners, reducing the licorice-like taste that often accompanies partially refined forms of stevia. Since stevia has practically no calories, mixing it with honey, sugar or even molasses is an excellent way to lower the caloric and sugar content of your favorite recipes. Stevia mixes particularly well with honey.

With weight watching and calorie counting practically having become a national pastime, virtually no-calorie stevia would seem to fill the bill as the perfect natural sweetener. But then again, we're not in Israel or China, South America or Japan where stevia is routinely used. You won't find it in handy packets on restaurant tables as you would in Tokyo, for instance.

The important thing to remember, however, is that stevia is now legally available here, and once you understand just "how sweet it is" — both in terms of taste and health benefits — you are empowered to make it a daily part of your regimen without having to wait for, or depend on, the commercial food industry to do it for you.

Sugar highs and lows

Even with all the negative publicity related to kids and sugar, many parents still find it easier to look the other way where candy or other sugary treats are concerned. One of the best reasons to incorporate stevia into your family's diet is to help your kids cut down on these ever present sugar-laden foods. (Of course we're hoping that you haven't started them on aspartame-laced products to accomplish that.)

A decade or so ago, refined sugar was given a bad rap by critics concerned about the relationship between sugar consumption and hyperactive and antisocial behavior, especially in children. As a result of developments like the "Twinkie defense" (used by the killer of San Francisco Mayor George Moscone and City Supervisor Harvey Milk), advertising firms and research labs got busy helping the sugar industry reinstate its upbeat "don't worry, be happy" premise.

An example of one such effort was a University of Wisconsin study involving 154 teenage males (134 of whom were considered delinquents). After feeding this group either a high-sugar or aspartame-sweetened breakfast cereal, the researchers soothingly concluded that "there was absolutely no evidence that sugar had any bad effects on any of the groups." They further noted that, among the kids with the worst behavioral problems, those who ate the sugar showed better performance (in a series of tests) than the ones in the aspartame group, and, in many of the nondelinquents, moods and behavior actually improved [1]

The University of Wisconsin study is just one in a slew of sugar-absolving research projects designed to attack the sugar-leads-to-aggression theories. While there may be no conclusive evidence linking a high-sugar diet to hyperactivity or criminal behavior, the major flaw in most of these studies is what they use to substitute for sugar — aspartame. Some aspartame critics claim that the artificial sweetener may be responsible for mood alteration and aggression. Many reports to the FDA of aspartame-adverse reactions involve a "change in mood quality or level."[2] But the researchers never suggested that this so-called 'placebo' (i.e., aspartame) might itself be altering the test results. The experiment, in fact, could well have been reversed, with aspartame being tested as an instigator of aggressive behavior and sugar used as the placebo.

Even if you don't feel particularly aggressive after a bowl of double sugar whammies, a common complaint after sugar indulgence (particularly on an empty stomach) is an uneasy feeling, which can be caused by the accompanying drop in blood sugar. If you are hypoglycemic (prone to low blood sugar), that drop can be severe, causing such symptoms as anxiety and sweating. Can you avoid these sugar blues by using stevia?

Beyond sweetening

In Paraguay, numerous medicinal benefits have been ascribed to stevia, dating back to the Indians and to Brazilian gauchos who describe a wonderful sense of well-being after drinking stevia-sweetened maté.[3]

While no conclusive studies have substantiated stevia's widely reported effect as a regulator of blood-sugar levels, a popular Paraguayan treatment for diabetes for more than 45 years has been a stevia tea concoction prepared from the leaves, stems and flowers.[4] Another Paraguayan remedy (for high blood-sugar levels) is a syrupy liquid made by boiling the leaves in water and adding the resulting thick solution to a variety of drinks.[5] (Some studies have indicated that stevia does not lower blood-sugar levels in the normal, i.e., nondiabetic, test animal.)

In Brazil, aside from a wide variety of approved food uses, stevia is permitted as a sugar substitute in dietetic products and in dental preparations,[6] and also has been widely used to improve digestion.[7]

Stevia's unique properties also make it ideal for toothpaste and mouthwash, since studies have indicated it might actually reduce cavities by retarding the growth of plaque in the mouth.[8]

The market value in naturally sweetened dental products has not gone unnoticed by manufacturers. An example is a new mouthwash, proudly touted as being "naturally sweetened with xylitol." Xylitol, which can be derived from birchwood, is now mostly produced from pulp-industry waste products.[9] In the United States xylitol was formerly used in chewing gums and some foods; however, such uses were voluntarily curtailed after several studies indicated it might cause tumors.[10] The fact that a product can claim to have "no artificial ingredients" has strong consumer appeal these days — enough so that some "natural" dental preparations have also resorted to sweetening their products with xylitol.

But you needn't wait for the big-name dental-products manufacturers to turn to stevia. A homemade mouthwash can easily be made by simply adding five or six drops of stevia concentrate to a small amount of water. You can also apply a stevia concentrate directly to the gums, massage and rinse. Stevia's antimicrobial properties are partly what make it so well suited to dental products. Tests have shown it can inhibit the growth of microbes such as streptococcus mutans.[11] Here again we can see the dramatic contrast between sugar, which promotes tooth decay, and stevia, which actually impedes it.

Water-based stevia concentrates are also marketed as skin care preparations, used to improve skin tone and treat blemishes. Before the Dietary Supplement Act permitted stevia sales in supplement form, consumers often purchased such "skin care" products, discarded the clay (which was ostensibly included to mix with the stevia), and used the stevia as a sweetener. With the approval of stevia as a dietary supplement, that charade is no longer necessary.

While stevia is certainly not a panacea (although in the People's Republic of China stevia tea is recommended for weight loss and for youthful vigor[12]), it has potentially important medicinal applications that have been ignored in this country. With the exception of limited research in the early 1950s by the National Institute of Arthritis and Metabolic Diseases,[13] most government efforts involving stevia have been convoluted maneuvers to keep it out of the marketplace altogether.

But then, stevia isn't the only traditionally recognized remedy to be treated with such official disdain. Acupuncture needles only recently received FDA reclassification as medical tools (they were formally considered experimental devices) — a classic example of how our supposedly "advanced" society often lags behind other, older cultures.

The difference in cooking with stevia

Stevia comes in many forms (see Chapter 6). One of the challenges in using these various forms of stevia in cooking and for beverages lies in finding just the right amount to suit your taste and recipe. If you're not accustomed to stevia's taste yet, you can mix it with another sweetener that has a distinct taste of its own (such as honey), creating a reduced-calorie version of the recipe. (Remember, stevia's synergistic effect with other sweeteners means you need much less of the other sweeteners than you think). If you're using stevia in a less refined form (such as crushed leaves), spices such as cinnamon and ginger can help mask any aftertaste. After using stevia for a while, you'll probably find yourself growing to love the taste it adds to foods and beverages.

One of the few recipes for which stevia is not recommended is in the making of yeast breads. Yeast needs to be "activated" by sugars, otherwise the bread won't rise. You'll also find that bakery products made with stevia won't brown like traditionally sweetened cookies or nonyeast breads. If you usually measure "doneness" by how brown something gets, instead, just stick a toothpick in the center to determine if it's sufficiently dry. As for cookies, we usually just test by sneaking a bite.

Still sweet after all these years

The term 'perennial' is not one that applies only to the stevia plant itself (when grown in the right climate, that is) but also to its sweetening powers.

James Duke, a former USDA botanist, has reported that leaves of "Paraguay's sweet herb" that he found in an old wrinkled envelope dated 1945 were still powerful enough to sweeten his coffee in 1986.[1] In a similar fashion, specimens of Stevia rebaudiana leaves preserved in a herbarium collection were found to have remained intensely sweet over a 60-year period.[2] Who says good things can't last?

Sweetener seems to be the hardest word

According to FDA officials, stevia's sweetening power is so "potent" that even in the low concentrations that would be used to flavor an herbal tea, for example, the agency just can't seem to "make that distinction" between its use as a flavoring agent and as a sweetener. Such a distinction was made, however, in the case of saccharin.

Since 1965, saccharin has been included in a growing list of largely synthetic flavoring ingredients considered to be "generally recognized as safe" (GRAS) by the flavor industry's trade coalition, the Flavor Extracts Manufacturers Association (FEMA).[1] Since FEMA deals solely with flavoring ingredients, how did this test-tube sweetener end up on the flavor industry's list of approved ingredients?

According to Richard Ford, former executive secretary of FEMA's Expert Panel, when FEMA first listed saccharin in 1965 as being "safe as used in flavorings," there was no reaction from the FDA, which "just ignored it." In 1978, FEMA reaffirmed saccharin for use in flavorings, again with no response from the agency. Although saccharin is not considered to be GRAS by the FDA, it still retains that status for use as a flavoring agent by virtue of the FEMA GRAS classification. And just what taste sensation is the flavor industry trying to achieve with saccharin's use? Whatever that is, says Ford, it's at "a level so low that the saccharin would impart no sweetness." Nor will you find saccharin on the label when used in this manner, as the word "flavoring" is all the FDA requires.[2]

Promises, promises

Because Brazil offers the potential of a huge soft-drink market, soda manufacturers couldn't have been more pleased when a 17-year ban on artificial sweeteners was lifted in 1988.[1]

While Coke, Pepsi and a number of Brazilian companies were anxiously awaiting the green light to flood the market with their sugar-free beverages, the Brazilian minister of health had other ideas.

His proposal: that only stevia-sweetened diet drinks be allowed in Brazil. As you can imagine, this idea encountered strong opposition from big companies with a lot to lose. (One company, Monsanto, had slated millions of dollars to construct a NutraSweet plant in the state of Sao Paulo.)[2]

After much protest, the proposed policy was dropped. In exchange for smooth government approval for the use of aspartame, cyclamates and saccharine in diet drinks, the Association of Soft Drink Manufacturers promised Brazil's Ministry of Health that its members would carry out studies to show how stevia could be included in their formulations.[3]

The results of those studies, which were supposed to have been produced by 1989, are long overdue. According to Dr. Howard Roberts, senior vice president of scientific and regulatory affairs for the National Soft Drink Association, it's not known what became of the promised studies, or even if they were done.

Dr. Roberts, however, does have a few things to say about both stevia and aspartame. In a paper he presented at the 1993 International Sweetener Colloquium, he describes some of stevia's uses in Japan, concluding that the "FDA has taken the position that extensive testing would be needed before its safety could be established." As for aspartame he notes: "The U.S. petition to expand permitted aspartame uses to include soft drinks was filed in 1982 and approved in 1983. The activists once again objected and pursued the issue all the way to the Supreme Court, where they finally lost the battle and gave up."

CHAPTER 6

A sweetener by any other name

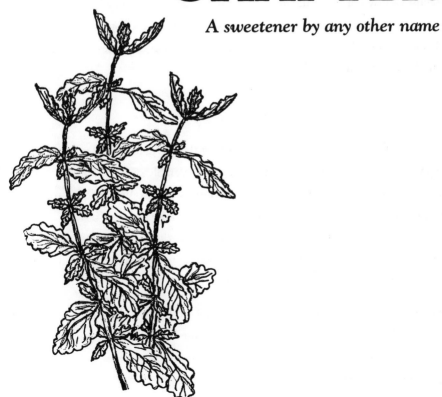

With stevia now permitted on the market as a dietary supplement, there are suddenly a variety of stevia products to choose from (even if none of them can officially be called sweeteners). Often, the very same formulation is labeled as both a dietary supplement and for other uses, such as skin care. Which stevia products you want to use will probably depend on the amount of sweetness required and the degree to which the particular recipe or beverage will benefit from the licorice-like taste that accompanies its less refined forms.

Fresh stevia leaves

This form of stevia is the herb in its most natural, unrefined state. A leaf picked from a stevia plant and chewed will impart an extremely sweet taste sensation reminiscent of licorice that lasts for quite a while. (In Bertoni's first official description of the stevia plant he noted that "a fragment of the leaf...suffices to keep the mouth sweet for an hour.")

For stevia to have a more practical application as a tea or sweetener, the leaves must be dried or put through an extraction process, which makes the sweet taste even more potent. Terrific-tasting stevia still comes from its native land, Paraguay, though China, Thailand, Canada and other countries also now grow stevia of comparable quality.

Dried leaves

For more of the flavor and sweet constituents of the stevia leaf to be released, drying and crushing is necessary. A dried leaf is considerably sweeter than a fresh one, and is the form of stevia used in brewing herbal tea. When added to herbal tea blends, amounts can be adjusted to provide more or less of a sweet taste. Lipton emphasized this difference in its GRAS petition to the FDA, stating that in the amounts the company proposed adding to its herbal tea blends, the stevia would impart only a "grassy, fresh taste."

Finely powdered or pulverized stevia leaf can be found both in bulk form and in tea bags. It has a greenish, leaf color and can be used as a flavor enhancer or sweetener in a wide variety of foods and beverages such as vegetables, coffee, applesauce and hot cereals.

Stevia extracts

The form in which stevia is primarily used as a sweetener in Japan is that of a white powdered extract (Body Ecology refers to it as "white stevia powder" in its stevia-sweetened recipes). In this form it is approximately 200 to 300 times sweeter then sugar (by weight). The sugar-type stevia packets found in many Japanese restaurants are bulked up with another substance (such as maltodextrin), since a much smaller amount of the extract itself is needed.

Around the world there are hundreds of patents for stevia extraction processes (the Japanese alone have over 150).

The sweet compounds in the stevia leaf are called glycosides. The most abundant glycoside is stevioside; the second is called rebaudioside. There are other sweet components of the leaf as well, but present in much smaller amounts. Rebaudiosides are considered to have a taste superior to steviosides, but since they make up a much smaller percentage of the leaf, most extraction processes make use of both compounds. However, there are some methods of extraction that are aimed at obtaining more of the better-tasting and sweeter rebaudioside-A compounds from the leaf.

Not all stevia extract powders are the same. The taste, sweetness and cost of the various white stevia powders will likely depend on their degree of refinement and the quality of the stevia plant used. You may find that some powders have more of an aftertaste. Some Canadian researchers have been developing a water extraction process for the sweet glycosides in the stevia leaf which they claim will be exceptionally sweet with practically no aftertaste (see box).

Since extracted stevia powder is so intensely sweet, we recommend that it be mixed with water and the solution used by the drop. Once mixed, this solution should be stored in the refrigerator. While the extracted powder is the most delicious form of stevia to use when replacing sugar or other sweeteners, any nutritional benefits (other than the elimination of sugar or harmful sugar substitutes from the diet) would probably be lost in the refining process.

Liquid concentrates

Liquid concentrates come in several forms. One method of distillation is to boil the leaves in water to achieve a water-based, syrup-like black liquid. Usually dispensed from a dropper-style bottle, it has a delicious taste that adds to the flavor of many foods, particularly hot beverages.

Another type of liquid concentrate is made by steeping the leaves in distilled water or water and grain alcohol. Some of these liquid preparations contain other ingredients such as chrysanthemum flowers, so if you only want pure ste-via leaf concentrate, be sure to check the label.

Stevia as a dietary supplement

Since stevia is now permitted entry into the U.S. only in the form of a dietary supplement, it's quite likely that all of the stevia or stevia-sweetened products you encounter will be labeled as such. A familiarity with the different forms in which stevia comes, however, can enable you to make the best use of each and to maximize the benefits you'll derive from this marvelous plant.

Stevia rebaudiana Bertoni:
The sweetest member of a big family tree

While over 200 different species of stevia grow around the world,[1] it's quite likely that Stevia rebaudiana may be the only one in its family that seriously worries the sweetener industry. Some of the other stevia species have even been described as having a bitter taste.[2]

Although none of the others have ever been studied or used as extensively as Stevia rebaudiana, many have reputations in the locales where they grow for possessing capabilities ranging from "preventing the fall of hair" to treating stomach aches, soothing burns and scratches, alleviating rheumatism, and even treating heart disease (Stevia cardiatica).[3]

Some of these traditional uses were described as far back as 1576 by Spanish physician Francisco Hernandez in his book, "Natural History of Plants of the New Spain."

Hot prospect in a cold climate

While stevia's historical roots may lie in Paraguay, its future direction could well be determined in Canada.

The Canadians first got into the act when two former University of Calgary chemistry professors devised a simple extraction process for stevioside that totally eliminates any aftertaste. They then teamed up with the Alberta Research Council in planning ways to make the effort commercially feasible.[1] The resulting venture: Royal Sweet International of Vancouver, a company that was formed for the sole purpose of developing this new stevia sweetener. This, in turn, has led to a joint project with Agriculture Canada (a government agency), which views stevia crops as a potential high-profit replacement for Canadian tobacco.[2]

While the use of refined stevia extracts as sugar replacements has not yet been approved by the Canadian government, there has never been a problem in buying imported stevia leaves at Canadian health food stores. In fact, a spokesman for the Canadian equivalent of the FDA (Health Canada) said it has no problem with stevia's use as a tea.

But as tasty as a cup of stevia tea may be, the big money for Royal Sweet International will have to come from its refined stevia powder, which will initially be targeted to the Asian market while North American approval is sought.

Whether it's Canadian naiveté about the goings-on here in the U.S. or just a 'whistling in the dark' attitude, Royal Sweet CEO William Barratt was quoted in the December 1995 edition of Technology Review as saying he believes that it "will take about three years for FDA approval" of its refined stevia product.[3]

Barratt also claims that the people at Royal Sweet have patented a new, improved stevia hybrid that's sweeter than any variety they've tasted so far.

CHAPTER 7
Home Sweet Home-Grown Stevia

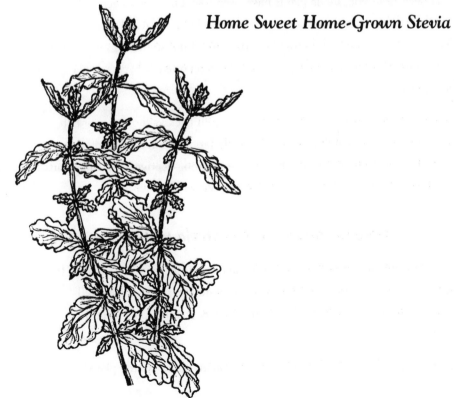

The feeling of satisfaction and self-sufficiency that comes from growing one's own produce — especially when done without the help of toxic chemicals — can be especially sweet for those who take a little extra time and effort to cultivate stevia as well. Stevia plants are remarkably easy to grow, and the bushy, velvety green leaves of the plant add an attractive note to any garden.

You need not be a South American planter to be a successful stevia grower. While the herb's native locale may make it appear somewhat exotic, it has proved to be quite adaptable and capable of being cultivated in climate zones as diverse as Florida and southern Canada.

True, home-grown stevia may lack the potency of refined white stevia extract, whose stevioside content generally ranges from 81 to 91 percent, as compared to a leaf level of approximately 12 percent. But it can provide you with a quantity of freshly harvested stevia 'tea leaves' to augment your supply of commercial stevia sweeteners.

Organic gardeners in particular should find stevia an ideal addition to their yield. Though nontoxic, stevia plants have been found to have insect-repelling tendencies. Their very sweetness, in fact, may be a kind of natural defense mechanism against aphids and other bugs that find it not to their taste. Perhaps that's why crop-devouring grasshoppers have been reported to bypass stevia under cultivation.

Then, too, raising stevia yourself, whether in your back yard or on your balcony, is another positive way you can personally (and quite legally) protest the wrongheaded government policies that have for so long deprived the American people of its benefits — a kind of contemporary Victory Garden.

How to start your own stevia patch

It would be difficult, at best, to start a stevia patch from scratch — that is, by planting seeds. Even if you could get them to germinate, results might well prove disappointing, since stevioside levels can vary greatly in plants grown from seed.

The recommended method is rather to buy garden-ready 'starter' plants, which, given stevia's 'growing' popularity, may well be obtainable from a nursery or herbalist in your area — provided you're willing to scout around a bit. If you're not, or are unsuccessful in locating any, there are at least three growers of high-quality stevia who will ship you as many baby plants as you'd like (see end of this chapter for details).

Keep in mind that not all stevia plants are created equal in terms of stevioside content, and, hence, sweetness. It's therefore a good idea to try to determine if the plants you're buying have been grown from cuttings whose source was high in stevioside.

Because tender young stevia plants are especially sensitive to low temperatures, it's important that you wait until the danger of frost is past and soil temperatures are well into the 50s and 60s before transplanting them into your garden.

Once you begin, it's best to plant your stevia in rows 20 to 24 inches apart, leaving about 18 inches between plants. Your plants should grow to a height of about 30 inches and a width of 18 to 24 inches.

The care and feeding of stevia

Stevia plants do best in a rich, loamy soil — the same kind in which common garden-variety plants thrive. Since the feeder roots tend to be quite near the surface, it is a good idea to add compost for extra nutrients if the soil in your area is sandy.

Besides being sensitive to cold during their developmental stage, the roots can also be adversely affected by excessive levels of moisture. So take care not to overwater them and to make sure the soil in which they are planted drains easily and isn't soggy or subject to flooding or "puddling."

Frequent light watering is recommended during the summer months. Adding a layer of compost or your favorite mulch around each stevia plant will help keep the shallow feeder roots from drying out.

Stevia plants respond well to fertilizers with a lower nitrogen content than the fertilizer's phosphoric acid or potash content. Most organic fertilizers (cow manure, fish emulsion, etc.) would work well since they release nitrogen slowly.

Gathering autumn stevia leaves

Harvesting should be done as late as possible, since cool autumn temperatures and shorter days tend to intensify the sweetness of the plants as they evolve into a reproductive state. While exposure to frost is still to be avoided, covering the plants during an early frost can give you the benefit of another few weeks' growth and more sweetness.

When the time does come to harvest your stevia, the easiest technique is to cut the branches off with pruning shears before stripping the leaves. As an extra bonus, you might also want to clip off the very tips of the stems and add them to your harvest, as they are apt to contain as much stevioside as do the leaves.

If you live in a relatively frost-free climate, your plants may well be able to survive the winter outside, provided you do not cut the branches too short (leaving about 4 inches of stem at the base during pruning). In that case, your most successful harvest will probably come in the second year. Three-year-old plants will not be as productive and, ideally, should be replaced with new cuttings.

In harsher climates, however, it might be a good idea to take cuttings that will form the basis for the next year's crop. Cuttings need to be rooted before planting, using either commercial rooting hormones or a natural base made from willow tree tips, pulverized into a slurry in your blender. After dipping the cuttings in such a preparation, the cuttings should be planted in a rooting medium for two to three weeks, giving the new root system a chance to form. They should then be potted — preferably in 4.5 inch pots — and placed in the sunniest and least drafty part of your home until the following spring.

Unlocking the sweetness in your harvest

Once all your leaves have been harvested you will need to dry them. This can be accomplished on a screen or net. (For a larger application, an alfalfa or grain drier can be used, but about the only way an average gardener might gain access to such a device is to borrow it from a friendly neighborhood farmer). The drying process is not one that requires excessive heat; more important is good air circulation. On a moderately warm fall day, your stevia crop can be quick dried in the full sun in about 12 hours. (Drying times longer than that will lower the stevioside content of the final product.) A home dehydrator can also be used, although sun drying is the preferred method.

Crushing the dried leaves is the final step in releasing stevia's sweetening power. This can be done either by hand or, for greater effect, in a coffee grinder or in a special blender for herbs. You can also make your own liquid stevia extract by adding a cup of warm water to 1/4 cup of dried, crushed stevia leaves. This mixture should set for 24 hours and then be refrigerated.

Growing stevia without land

Just because you live within the confines of an apartment or condominium doesn't mean you can't enjoy the benefits of stevia farming. This versatile plant can be grown either in pots on your balcony or any sunny spot, or else in a hydroponic unit. Stevia plants also do quite well in "container gardens." A 10" to 12" diameter container filled with a lightweight growing mix is an ideal size for each plant. A little mulch on the top will help retain the moisture in the shallow root zone. A properly fertilized hydroponic unit or container garden can provide you with as much stevia as an outdoor garden, if not more.

Sources for mail-order stevia plants

The **Herbal Advantage** is a Missouri herb supplier offering 2 1/4" pot size stevia plants ready for planting in your garden. For information and prices, call 800-753-9929, or write to them at Rte. 3, Box 93, Rogersville, MO 65742.

Richter's Herbs, a Canadian concern, offers plants in 2 1/2" pots via courier to customers in the U.S. and Canada. For information and prices, you can call (905) 640-6677 or fax them at (905) 640-6641 or write them at 357 Highway 47, Goodwood, Ontario L0C-1A0

Well Sweep Herb Farm is another source offering plants in 3" pots either via mail order or to customers who stop by. It is located at 205 Mt. Bethel Road, Port Murray, NJ 07865 or can be reached at (908) 852-5390

CONCLUSION

Getting stevia on the market in the form of a dietary supplement has been an event of critical significance in making the benefits of this marvelous herb available to the American public. But the battle is far from won. As of this writing, the wall erected by the FDA is still very much in place. It is difficult to know how much more effort — or even just what sort of effort — will be required for stevia to achieve the kind of alternative sweetener status in the U.S. that it has been accorded in other countries.

In an August 1996 interview with The Fresno Bee on the subject of stevia, FDA spokesman Arthur Whitmore commented that it's one thing to allow individuals to use a product and something else entirely to allow it to be added to the general food supply. He added that just because something is natural doesn't automatically mean it's safe, citing the example of hemlock, a deadly poison.

His innuendo is but one more clear indication that the FDA is not yet ready to abandon its campaign of tarring stevia with the same brush it uses for dangerous substances. And, indeed, such disparaging references, bearing as they do an official FDA stamp of disapproval, might well serve their purpose in scaring off the uninformed.

In reality, of course, no one is claiming that stevia is safe by virtue of being natural. It's naturalness, however, has enabled people to use it for centuries, and it is this test of time — amply supported by modern scientific research — that permits us to say that stevia is a truly beneficial substance that can be used without fear of adverse consequences. Clearly the barrier to its approval is not one raised by scientific concerns, but rather by commercial concerns, augmented by bureaucratic intransigence.

Until such time as stevia can be used without restraint in the general food supply, and calorie-conscious (or diabetic) consumers can have a choice between stevia-sweetened products and those laced with aspartame or saccharin, the public will still be denied its full rights to a healthful dietary lifestyle.

That time will come sooner or later — but come it will. The timing depends on the pressure brought to bear on our political and regulatory bodies. Writing to your congressional representative is one approach, of course, but that is only a first step. What's most important is to spread the word, and to keep this grass-roots movement growing.

Our political system was not intended to be dominated by unyielding bureaucrats or corporate lobbyists — but it will be if we let it. It is only by maintaining the momentum for change, individually and collectively, that we can effectively counter their influence — and help the American public find a healthful alternative way to satisfy its sweet tooth.

COOKING WITH STEVIA

Before making stevia-sweetened dishes part of your recipe repertoire, there are some important things to keep in mind.

First, stevia cannot be substituted for sugar on a cup-for-cup basis. Because refined stevia powder can be 200-300 times sweeter than sugar, just 1/2 teaspoon of white stevia powder equals approximately 1 cup of sugar in sweetening power. We say *approximately* because different brands of stevia vary in sweetness.

Stevia is delicious in almost any recipe using fruit or dairy products. However, it presents a challenge when used for baking. Sugar lends special properties to cookies and cakes that are not present in stevia. Sugar enhances the tenderness and the moistness of flour products. It provides bulk and leavening to the dough. In yeast products the sugars serve as food for the yeast. The volume of many cakes depends upon creaming the shortening (butter) with sugar and eggs. There is no doubt in our minds that once stevia is discovered by our best-known food chemists and professional chefs, solutions will be found to make stevia work with flour products too. Until then, the recipes that follow are great examples of how to use stevia. We urge you to do what we've done: experiment.

Our Body Ecology chefs are always creating new recipes. We are currently developing a cookbook using 50 delicious stevia-sweetened recipes. Look for **Stevia The Miracle No Calorie Sweetener** (available summer 1997).

Try stevia in teas, soda drinks, shakes, puddings, candy, ice cream, cheese cakes, pies and even tofu or soymilk desserts. Once again, it is especially delicious with fruit and dairy flavors.

Stevia can be combined with a variety of natural sugars such as honey, maple syrup, molasses, rice syrup, barley malt and fructose, greatly reducing the amount of sugar in a recipe. This can be a valuable aid for anyone (especially parents) not wanting to completely eliminate sugar, but trying to minimize its use.

ONE WORD OF CAUTION:

The Body Ecology Diet has earned a reputation for being the ideal way to eat for anyone with candidiasis, chronic fatigue, cancer, AIDS, M.S. and many other immune disorders. It is important to stress that many of the following recipes were developed for someone *who does not have an immune disorder* and simply wants to experiment with stevia and take that first step toward a healthier lifestyle by eliminating sugar (or artificial sweeteners) from their diet. Since many of these recipes contain dairy products and/or fruits, these recipes are **not yet suitable** for you.

ANOTHER TIP:

Sometimes working with the white powder is a little difficult since stevia powder is so intensely sweet. A liquid concentrate solution may be more convenient, especially for sweetening beverages. We recommend you keep both on hand.

To make a liquid concentrate solution :
Add 1 teaspoon white stevia powder to 3 tablespoons of filtered water. Pour into a small dropper bottle and refrigerate.

Look for

STEVIA: The Miracle No Calorie Sweetener
Body Ecology's newest cookbook (available summer 1997)

STEVIA RECIPES

KEY:

Fine for occasional use for level one B.E.D.ers.

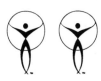

Okay for occasional use if in level two of B.E.D. After symptoms are gone, inner ecosystem is restored and you have begun to successfully add in new foods...especially those mentioned in Chapter 21, *How to Reintroduce Other Healthy Foods Into Your Diet* (see ***The Body Ecology Diet***).

CREAMY RICE PUDDING©

Ingredients:
1 cup basmati rice
1 cup heavy cream
2 cups + 1 cup water
1/4 tsp. white stevia powder
1/2 cup raisins
1/2 cup shredded coconut
1 tsp. cinnamon
1/2 tsp. nutmeg
1/2 tsp. sea salt

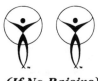

(If No Raisins)

1. To Cook Rice: In a medium saucepan, bring two cups of water to a boil. Add 1/2 tsp. sea salt and one cup basmati rice. Bring to a second boil, cover, reduce heat to low and cook 30 minutes until rice is tender.
2. Combine cream, stevia, cinnamon, nutmeg, raisins, coconut and remaining one cup of water with rice. Mix well.
3. Place rice mixture in a casserole dish and sprinkle with cinnamon. Bake at 350° for 25 - 30 minutes or until pudding is firm. Serve warm.

BANANA/SQUASH CHEESE CAKE©

Ingredients:
2-8 oz. packages of cream cheese, room temperature
4 cups butternut squash, cooked, peeled and seeded
4 eggs
2 Tbsp. non-alcoholic vanilla flavoring
1 tsp. Spice Hunter® Sweet Spice Blend
1/4 tsp. white stevia powder
1 cup Westbrae® ginger snap cookies, crushed in blender
1/2 stick unsalted butter
3 bananas

1. Preheat oven to 400°. Bake butternut squash whole for 1 to 1-1/2 hours, turning once until evenly soft. Remove from oven, slice, peel and remove seeds. Allow to cool.
2. **Crust:** Crumble the ginger snap cookies in blender until the crumbs are finely chopped. Add butter and mix well.
3. Butter the bottom of a cheesecake pan and line the sides with parchment paper. Place crumbs in the bottom of the pan and pat smooth.
4. **Filling:** Combine butternut squash, cream cheese, bananas, eggs, stevia, Sweet Spice Blend and vanilla flavoring. Blend until smooth. Pour into crust.
5. Place cheesecake pan in a larger pan filled with water to 3/4 of the height of the cheesecake pan. Bake for 1 hour.
6. Allow to cool and serve.

BITTERSWEET CHOCOLATE CANDY©

Ingredients:
8 oz. Baker's® unsweetened bittersweet chocolate,
2 1/2 sticks unsweetened butter, room temperature
12 oz. heavy cream
1 Tbsp. + 1 tsp. non-alcoholic vanilla flavoring
1 Tbsp. + 1 tsp. non-alcoholic brandy flavoring
1/2 tsp. white stevia powder

1. Over medium-low heat, slowly melt bittersweet chocolate in a double boiler. (Steam should be rising off the water...not a full boil.) Stir in pieces of butter until smooth and glossy. Take care not to lower the temperature of the mixture by adding butter too quickly.
2. Add cream, vanilla flavoring, brandy flavoring and stevia. Stir well until smooth and glossy. Adjust sweetness by adding more stevia if desired.
3. Refrigerate until mixture becomes solid.
4. Make balls (about the size of grapes) by scooping with melon baller or spoon. Dip your utensil in hot water frequently to make process easier.
5. Refrigerate again, and once chilled, roll balls into your favorite topping (coconut, walnuts, etc).

VANILLA ICE-CREAM©

Ingredients:
2 egg yolks
1/2 tsp. white stevia powder
2 cups cream
1 cup milk
2 tsp. non-alcoholic vanilla flavoring

1. In a blender, whip all ingredients very well.
2. Chill the whipped ingredients.
3. Pour chilled mixture into your ice-cream maker and follow directions for freezing.

Variation: Add fruit, carob or chocolate chips or nuts once mixture is semi-frozen, then complete freezing process. For a special treat garnish with **Carob Fudge Sauce** and **Sweet Whipped Cream Topping.**

CAROB FUDGE SAUCE©

Ingredients:
8 oz. heavy cream
1 tsp. non-alcoholic vanilla flavoring
1-1/4 cup unsweetened carob chips
1/4 tsp. white stevia powder (or to taste)

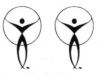

1. In a medium size saucepan, warm the cream over low heat.
2. Slowly adding carob chips, stir frequently until chips begin to melt.
3. Continue adding chips and then stevia powder until mixture is smooth. Remove from heat, let cool slightly then add vanilla flavoring.
4. Check sweetness of carob sauce and add more stevia if desired.
5. Delicious served over puddings, ice-creams or whenever a carob sauce is desired.

CHOCOLATE SAUCE©

To make a chocolate sauce follow the above instructions and substitute one square unsweetened (bittersweet) chocolate, then add more stevia to achieve desired sweetness. Non-alcoholic flavorings such as vanilla, orange, mint and coffee enhance the chocolate/stevia flavor. Grated orange and lemon peel are excellent flavor enhancers too.

SWEET WHIPPED CREAM TOPPING©

Ingredients:
1 pint of heavy whipping cream
1/8 tsp. white stevia powder

1. Place heavy cream in mixing bowl and whip with electric mixer or hand whisk until thickening occurs.
2. Sift stevia into cream and continue whipping.
3. Store in refrigerator in an airtight container.

SWEET CORN MUFFINS©

Ingredients:
1 cup Fern Brown Rice Baking Mix®
1 egg, slightly beaten
2 Tbsp. Body Ecology's Coconut Oil™, melted
1 Tbsp. liquid stevia concentrate* (see below)
3/4 cup milk
1-2 cups corn, fresh or frozen

1. Preheat oven to 400˚.
2. In a blender, add egg, milk and corn. Blend, then add coconut oil and stevia concentrate.
3. Add baking mix and blend until slightly lumpy.
4. Pour into lightly oiled muffin pan and bake for 20 minutes. (We use mini-muffin pans.)

To make a liquid concentrate solution:
Add 1 teaspoon white stevia powder to 3 tablespoons of filtered water. Pour into a small dropper bottle and refrigerate.

YUMMY KEFIR SHAKE©

Ingredients:
8 oz. plain kefir*
white stevia powder (to taste)
Non-alcoholic flavoring (vanilla, blueberry, peach, banana, strawberry, lemon, lime, orange coconut or almond)

1. Using an electric blender, blend all ingredients.
2. Pour into decorative glasses and enjoy.

To further enrich this nourishing drink:
> add unrefined organic oils such as flax seed, borage seed, Body Ecology's Essential Balance™), lactose free whey, lecithin granules and probiotics (friendly bacteria). Adding a 10 oz. package of organic frozen fruit (strawberries, blueberries or raspberries) is especially popular with children.

*Kefir is a cultured, enzyme-rich food chock full of friendly micro-organisms that help balance your "inner ecosystem." More nutritious and therapeutic than yogurt, it supplies complete protein, essential minerals, and valuable B vitamins. Read Body Ecology's *The Magic of Kefir: An Ancient Food for Modern Maladies* to learn more about kefir.

RECIPES USING
UNREFINED STEVIA

STEVIA APPLE CINNAMON SAUCE

To a serving of unsweetened applesauce add 1/8 of a teaspoon of powdered stevia leaves or 3 to 6 drops of liquid (black) concentrate (Wisdom of the Ancients®). Add cinnamon (and ginger powder if you like) to taste.

COFFEE AND TEA

To add a unique taste (as well as to sweeten) coffee and tea, you can use these forms of unrefined stevia.

*   To use the *liquid (black) concentrate*, add 3 to 6 drops in a cup of coffee or tea.

*   *Powdered leaves* can be sprinkled on top of ground coffee before brewing. Use about 1/2 teaspoon for 10 to 12 cups.

*   Of course, the *white stevia powder liquid concentrate* can also be used drop by drop to taste.

NOTES

CHAPTER 2:   Centuries-old appeal and contemporary intrigue

1. Elton Johnson, "Stevioside, Naturally" presentation to the Calorie Control Council, November, 1990.

2. Arent, Fox, Kintner, Plotkin and Kahn: GRAS petition to the FDA on behalf of the American Herbal Products Association: 18, April 23, 1992.

3. Ibid.

4. Dr. Moises Bertoni: KAA HE-HE, Its nature and its properties, Paraguayan Scientific Annals: 10, December, 1905

5. Herb Research Foundation: Supplement to GRAS Affirmation Petition 2G0390, Stevia rebaudiana Bertoni: 3

6. Republic of Paraguay, Ministry of Agriculture and Livestock General Planning Division: Questions to be answered about "Stevia."

7. D.D. Soejarto, et al., Potential Sweetening Agents of Plant Origin, Field Search for Sweet-Tasting Stevia Species: Economic Botany, 77, 1983

8. George S. Brady, American Trade Commissioner, Memo for Latin American Division: August 31, 1921

9. Report, Official Public Laboratory of Hamburg, 1913

10. Dr. Hewitt G. Fletcher, Jr., The Sweet Herb of Paraguay: Chemurgic Digest, 18, July/August, 1955

11. Hideo Fujita, Tomoyoshi Edahiro, Safety and Utilization of Stevia Sweetener

12. A. Douglas Kinghorn, Ph.D.: Food Ingredient Safety Review, Stevia rebaudiana leaves, 8, March 16, 1992

13. Dr. Laura Fracchia, Dr. Miguel Gonzalez Moreira, Memorandum, National Institute of Technology and Standardization, Asuncion, Paraguay: Bibliographical Report on the Stevia Rebaudiana Bertoni, 5, August 27, 1991

14. Letter to Marsha W. Gardner, McKenna & Cuneo, from Alan M. Rulis, Director, Division of Food and Color Additives, Center for Food Safety and Applied Nutrition, April 22, 1992

CHAPTER 3: What's wrong with Stevia?

1. Supplement to GRAS Affirmation Petition No. 4G0406: Stevia rebaudiana Bertoni (Stevia Leaf) for Use in Flavored and Herbal Teas, Volume I of II, Thomas J. Lipton Company, 45, February 3, 1995

2. Interview with Dr. Joseph Kuc, July, 1995

3. Interview with Dr. Joseph Kuc, July, 1995

4. Ibid 2 at 43

5. Professor Mauro Alvarez, Department of Pharmacy and Pharmacology, Maringa, Parana, Brazil: Contraceptive Effect of Stevia and its Sweetening Components

6. Ibid 2 at 46

7. Interview with Dr. David Hattan

8. Interview with Dr. Alan Rulis

9. Interview with Dr. George Pauli

10. Interview with Dr. Alan Rulis

11. A. Douglas Kinghorn, Ph.D.: Food Ingredient Safety Review, Stevia rebaudiana leaves, 12, March 16, 1992

12. Ibid at 21

BOXES IN CHAPTER 3

No sweet talk allowed

1. Stuart Pape, Could Your Food Product be a Dietary Supplement?: Prepared Foods, 25, February, 1995

2. Ibid

3. Revision of Import Alert # 45-06, Automatic Detention of Stevia Leaves, Extract of Stevia Leaves, and Foods Containing Stevia, September 18, 1995

What about Steviol?

1. K.C. Phillips: Stevia: Steps in Developing a New Sweetener, Keith Phillips & Associates, Newbury, Berkshire, UK

CHAPTER 4: What's wrong with the FDA?

1. James S. Turner: *The Chemical Feast*, 107 - 108

2. Ibid at 109

3. Peter Barton Hutt: Approval of Food Additives in the United States: A Bankrupt System, 43 - 44

4. William Greider: *Who Will Tell The People: The Betrayal of American Democracy*, 54 -55

5. Ibid 1 at 107

CHAPTER 5: A craving for sweets

1. Jean Carper: Food - *Your Miracle Medicine*, 303

2. Memorandum, Department of Health and Human Services: Adverse reactions associated with aspartame consumption, April 1, 1993

3. Third Brazilian Seminar on Stevia rebaudiana Bertoni, July 3 - 4, 1986

4. A. Douglas Kinghorn, Ph.D.: Food Ingredient Safety Review, Stevia rebaudiana leaves, 6, March 16, 1992

5. Ibid at 7

6. Ibid at 14

7. Daniel B. Mowrey, Ph.D., Life with Stevia: How Sweet It Is, 10

8. Ibid at 9

9. Ruth Winter: A Consumer's Dictionary of Food Additives, 420

10. Chris Lecos, Fructose: Questionable Diet Aid: FDA Consumer, March, 1980

11. Ibid 7 at 9

12. Ibid 4 at 13

13. Dr. Hewitt G. Fletcher, Jr., The Sweet Herb of Paraguay: Chemurgic Digest, 7, July/August, 1955

BOXES IN CHAPTER 5

Still sweet after all these years

1. James A. Duke, Stevia Rebaudiana: The Business of Herbs, 4, November/December 1986

2. A.D. Kinghorn, D.D. Soefarto, Current Status of Stevioside as a Sweetening Agent for Human Use, Economic and Medicinal Plant Research, 1985

Sweetener seems to be the hardest word

1. Recent Progress in the Consideration of Flavoring Ingredients Under the Food Additives Amendment, III. GRAS Substances: Food Technology, 294, February, 1965

2. Interview with Richard Ford

Promises, promises

1. Rik Turner, Paula M. Block: Brazil's Stevia Courts Bottlers, Chemical Week, 9, June 22, 1988

2. Ibid

3. Brazil Okays Diet Soft Drinks: Chemical Week, 44, August 3, 1988

BOXES IN CHAPTER 6

Stevia rebaudiana Bertoni: sweetest member of a big family tree

1. D.D. Soefarto, et al., Potential Sweetening Agents of Plant Origin.ll., Field Search for Sweet-Tasting Stevia Species: Economic Botany, 71-79, 1983

2. D.D. Soejarto, et al., Ethnobotanical Notes on Stevia: Botanical Museum Leaflets, Winter, 1983

3. Ibid

Hot prospect in a cold climate

1. A Sweet Future for Stevia: Alberta Report, June 5, 1995

2. Ibid

3. The Perfect Sweetener?: Technology Review, November/December, 1995

INDEX

G

G.D. Searle, 16

generally recognized as safe
    FEMA GRAS, 57
    history of, 43
    self-determination of, 28

Germany, 17, 25, 26

glycosides, 61

GRAS, 5, 28, 29, 30, 43, 44, 46, 57, 60

Greider, William, 46

Guarani Indians, 23, 27

H

Hattan, Dr. David, 30, 36

Hayes, Authur Hull, 16

Health Canada, 56

Herb Research Foundation, 24, 35

Herbalgram, 35

high fructose corn syrup, 14

Hoechst Celanese Corp., 17

honey, 3, 8, 14, 51, 54

Hutt, Peter Barton, 44

hypoglycemic, 35, 36, 52

I

Internet, 45

Israel, 26, 51

J

Japan, 7, 9, 11, 25, 26, 38, 51, 58, 61

Japanese
    discovery of stevia, 26
    Japanese Ministry of Health and Welfare, 40
    safety studies, 38
    stevia patents, 61
    uses of stevia, 26, 38, 51

S